SUPER IMMUNITY FOODS

A COMPLETE PROGRAM TO BOOST WELLNESS, SPEED RECOVERY, AND KEEP YOUR BODY STRONG

FRANCES SHERIDAN GOULART, CCN

Mc
Graw
Hill

New York Chicago San Francisco Lisbon London Madrid Mexico City
Milan New Delhi San Juan Seoul Singapore Sydney Toronto

Library of Congress Cataloging-in-Publication Data

Goulart, Frances Sheridan.
    Super immunity foods : a complete program to boost wellness, speed recovery, and keep
your body strong / by Frances Sheridan Goulart.
       p.   cm.
    ISBN 13: 978-0-07-159882-8 (alk. paper)
    ISBN 10: 0-07-159882-0 (alk. paper)
    1. Nutrition.   2. Functional foods.   3. Cookery (Natural foods)   I. Title.

RA784.G682   2009
613.2—dc22   2008047200

1 2 3 4 5 6 7 8 9 10 11 12 13 14 15 16 17 18 19 20 21 22 23 24   FGR/FGR 0 9

ISBN 978-0-07-159882-8
MHID   0-07-159882-0

Interior design by Monica Baziuk

McGraw-Hill books are available at special quantity discounts to use as premiums and sales
promotions or for use in corporate training programs. To contact a representative, please visit the
Contact Us pages at www.mhprofessional.com.

The information contained in this book is intended to provide helpful and informative material
on the subject addressed. It is not intended to serve as a replacement for professional medical
advice. Any use of the information in this book is at the reader's discretion. The author and
publisher disclaim any and all liability arising directly or indirectly from the use or application of
any information contained in this book.

This book is printed on acid-free paper.

To

My intrepid agent, Evelyn Fazio, and

my oh, so understanding editor, Sarah Pelz.

And as always, my backup crew: Ron, Sean, and Steffan.

—

CONTENTS

.... ❧ ....

INTRODUCTION

APPLES, ORANGES, AND ANTIBIOTICS

.... ❧ ....

Understanding Immunity

"IN THE NEXT TEN years," says Katherine Tucker, Ph.D., of the Tufts University Friedman School of Nutrition Science and Policy, "individuals will go to their doctors, have their genetics analyzed, and be told, for example, that fish oil can help reduce their risk of heart disease and Alzheimer's." But there's no need to wait for the science of nutrigenetics to hit its stride—you have all the tools for taking your health into your own hands at your local grocery store. With the help of this book, you can start eating all the super foods that boost immunity so you can stay fit and healthy, starting with your very next meal.

Super Immunity Foods: What, Where, and Why

....

And what are those super foods? Berries, tree fruits, root vegetables, leafy greens, and grains; plus the ancient healing food, yogurt; and vegetables from the sea, such as kelp and dulse. According to a study by researchers at the Harvard School of Public Health, people who consume eight or more servings of fruits and vegetables a day may reduce their risk of cardiovascular disease by more than 20 percent compared to those eating only three servings a day. Even better, the risk and incidence of every other major disease, including diabetes, cancer, and arthritis, also declines as the intake of red, green, blue, white, and brown foods goes up. Red foods, such as tomatoes and cherries, provide the antioxidants lycopene and anthocyanins for a healthy heart and clean arteries, while yellow and orange foods provide vitamin C and bioflavonoids for healthy vision and lowered cancer risk. Blue and purple foods are rich in plant nutrients called phenolics for diabetes control and antiaging benefits, while white foods like garlic and potatoes help lower cholesterol and control respiratory disease.

Every whole food dishes up something important, but the twenty-five foods that top the list and do the most to support immunity are apples, berries, broccoli, carrots, citrus fruits, dark leafy greens, green food powders, figs and dates, garlic, flaxseed, legumes, oats, olives, herbs and spices, mushrooms, potatoes, sea vegetables, squash, tomatoes, soy foods, nuts and seeds, whole grains, and yogurt.

Apples Versus Antibiotics: More Reasons to Eat Super Immunity Foods

....

In addition to improved health and vitality, there are a number of reasons for taking a proactive approach to your immunity and well-being. From commonly prescribed drugs to pollutants in the air and water (not to mention stress!), you have plenty of reasons to take your health into your own hands with super immunity foods.

An Epidemic of Antibiotics

Reaching for an apple, some oatmeal, or an herb before you have to start taking an antibiotic is smart. Antibiotics are now the leading cause of adverse drug reactions in the United States and the cause of often deadly strains of resistant bacteria. In addition, antibiotics are commonly overprescribed. Even though, for example, most sore throats are viral and not bacterial in nature (therefore, resistant to antibiotics), 73 percent of viral sore throats are often treated with an antibiotic prescription, according to a yearlong study by the U.S. Food and Drug Administration Center for Drug Evaluation and Research.

While super pills may help with super infections caused by bacteria, drugs such as penicillin and sulfur drugs can lower your resistance even as they help you fight back. In the process of killing those bad bugs, antibiotics deplete a wide spectrum of nutrients that are the foundation for immunity, including vitamin C, iron, zinc, and most of the B vitamins, plus bone-building vitamin K, calcium, and magnesium. In addition, antibiotics wipe out your good bacteria, so they are best used only when truly necessary—and even better, avoid them altogether with super immunity nutrition.

The Truth About Water from the Tap

Even those of us who don't take antibiotics intentionally are getting them unintentionally. In recent studies, every body of water that the United States tested for drug residues contained trace amounts of antibiotics from human waste and from animal farms that use antibiotics as growth promoters. Tap water may also be contaminated with trace amounts of a rocket fuel chemical called perchlorate (also used in fireworks and safety flares) that can disrupt thyroid function and cause cancer in adults and mental retardation in newborns, according to the Environmental Working Group in a 2005 study.

Toxins in our waters all lower immunity. According to researchers at the University of Texas, simply taking showers and using the dishwasher liberate trace amounts of chlorine. These are then inhaled, releasing by-products such as dioxin, which according to the Environmental Protection Agency is 300,000 times more potent a carcinogen than DDT.

Bad Habits Break Down Immunity

Immunity also breaks down in response to our deliberate bad habits. According to a recent World Health Report, unhealthy diets, inactivity, and tobacco use are the main culprits behind chronic ailments that cause 60 percent of all premature deaths from cancer, heart disease, and cancer each year. The World Health Organization (WHO) estimates that if this trend continues, new cancer cases worldwide may increase by 50 percent.

Smoking is bad, and the use of recreational drugs isn't any better. Did you know that delta-9-tetrahydrocannabinol (THC), the most active component in marijuana, depresses the immune response and makes the white blood cells in the respiratory immune center or elsewhere 35 to 40 percent less effective?

You Are Only as Healthy as the Foods You Eat

Eating defensively to build resistance is an art. The discrepancy between who we are and what we put in our bodies using our knives and forks, as critics have observed, has laid the groundwork for the current epidemic of illness and disease. According to USDA nutrition information between 1973 and 1997, nutrient levels in all fresh vegetables declined significantly. Calcium levels in broccoli alone dropped 53 percent.

In not so-fresh foods, things are even less nourishing. Besides everything else wrong with them, 70 percent of all processed foods contain gene-altered ingredients, whose long-term risks are unknown. Processed foods, it turns out, are also delivery systems for residues of the flame-retardant polybrominated diphenyl ethers (PBDEs), which bioaccumulate in the body with unknown health consequences. Nine out of ten common grocery products contain them, including cheese, butter, eggs, and fish.

According to the Pesticide Action Network, nine out of ten people also carry traces of the insecticide TCP as part of their body burden, along with breakdown products of DDT, which are used in growing nonorganic and especially imported fruits and vegetables. In addition, many of these chemicals can cause cancer, disrupt hormone systems, adversely affect fertility, and weaken the immune system.

A Breath of Not-So-Fresh Air: Environmental Pollutants and Everyday Stress

Other factors that contribute to decreased immunity include exposure to a wide and increasing range of pollutants in the air, water, and soil. There's a wide range of other immunity-busting triggers, from mercury amalgam dental fillings, to an underactive thyroid, to allergies, to exposure to low-level radiation from cell phones and other devices. Even a mental outlook that is more down than up can do in your immunity.

The First Step to Super Immunity

Food can help—the right foods. That means a lot more fruits and vegetables than most of us eat. Elephants put away more than 6,000 cabbages, apples, carrots, and other vegetables a year. All *you* have to do is put away a minimum of five to nine servings of fruits and vegetables a day—focusing on the super immunity foods—to boost your immunity. It's still a tall order, judging by how far most of us fall from the mark.

But it's worth the effort.

Did you know . . .

▶ the older you get, the less heart-essential coenzyme Q10 you have? Not so good, since 95 percent of the energy produced by the body depends on this electron transport chemical, making it important to eat more and more energy-producing greens, grains, and beans.

▶ beans or grains that are refined or processed have a higher glycemic index? This means they raise your blood sugar higher per serving than their natural counterparts, leading to weight gain.

▶ raw mushrooms contain potentially carcinogenic compounds that are destroyed by cooking?

▶ a cup of the ancient grain quinoa supplies as much protein as a glass of milk—and more calcium?

And how about conventional kitchen wisdom? Is it true, for example, what they say about an apple a day? And what about the anticancer qualities of soybeans?

Building immunity aside, what do you do if you already have a disorder or condition that is the result of impaired defenses? How do you eat your way out of cancer, heart disease, allergies, or everyday headaches caused by stress?

This book delivers all those answers. Once you know what foods you've got to eat, you will get easy but effective recipes to go with them, plus menu plans and strategies for putting the whole program together.

A journey of a thousand miles may begin with a single step, but our journey of twenty-five foods begins with a simple quiz.

Super Immunity Quiz

Is your immunity in the red, the black, or the twilight zone? Test it out, answering with a yes or no. Do you . . .

_____ **1.** *have more than two colds or infections a year?*
_____ **2.** *smoke?*
_____ **3.** *drink soda, coffee, or alcohol almost daily?*
_____ **4.** *drink fluoridated water?*

_____ 5. *get less than six hours of undisturbed sleep most nights?*

_____ 6. *have dark circles or puffiness under your eyes?*

_____ 7. *have more than 10 pounds to lose?*

_____ 8. *use more than three prescription drugs regularly?*

_____ 9. *take recreational drugs regularly?*

_____ 10. *live near an interstate or heavily trafficked area?*

_____ 11. *make processed foods more than 50 percent of your diet?*

_____ 12. *rarely buy organic foods?*

_____ 13. *eat fast foods more than once a week?*

_____ 14. *drink less than eight glasses of water daily?*

_____ 15. *feel fatigued often or all the time?*

_____ 16. *have constipation, diarrhea, or both more than once a month?*

_____ 17. *crave salty, fatty, or sugary foods?*

_____ 18. *rarely take nutritional supplements?*

_____ 19. *have unstable emotions or frequent headaches?*

_____ 20. *have bad breath or irritated skin?*

_____ 21. *exercise less than two hours a week?*

_____ 22. *use no stress-management strategies (e.g., meditation, yoga, relaxation therapies)?*

_____ 23. *wear commercial nail polish products or nonorganic hygiene and beauty products?*

_____ 24. *use a cell phone without a headset or radiation-blocking device?*

_____ 25. *have few social ties to friends and community?*

Count the number of yes answers.

SCORING:
Low immunity: 15–23
Fair immunity: 10–14
Good immunity: 5–9
Excellent immunity: 0–4

Want a more scientific immunity test? You can get your C-reactive protein (CRP) tested. This protein in the blood becomes elevated when one or more of the immune systems is overactive. Overactivity is a marker for disease. High levels of CRP can signal pending high blood pressure or stroke, Alzheimer's, macular degeneration, or colon, prostate, or other cancers. Even better, ask your doctor for a high-sensitivity CRP (hs-CRP) test to determine your true immunity level.

THE BODY'S SIX
IMMUNE CENTERS

"OUR OWN PHYSICAL BODY possesses a wisdom which we who inhabit it lack," observed author Henry Miller. The immune system, in its own wisdom, is, functionally speaking, not one system but several—six, in fact.

Immune cells defending us from harm keep company with one another in an interlocking round-the-clock system of biotelepathy throughout the body. It's the equivalent of having a squad of bodyguards always on call but positioned according to purpose. Thus your heart and arteries are protected by the defensive cellular team in your cardiovascular center, while the liver, kidney, and bladder, more concerned with detoxification and cleansing, call up a different but equally vigilant squad of cells and cellular defenses as needed.

Different organs, structures, and substances are all involved. In general, what causes immunity to stumble and leave us vulnerable to disease is the overactivity of one or more of the body's six immune centers. In response to exposure to toxins, your overactive white blood cells begin to attack neurons in the brain (causing aging, Alzheimer's, or dementia, for example), or the lining of the arteries (causing coronary or arterial disease), or the cartilage in the joints (causing osteoarthritis). And we all have our combinations of strengths and weaknesses that make us unique—strong heart, weak knees; bad bones, good digestion; bad back, good mind—so we are defended and fight back in uniquely different ways.

Weakening of the immune centers or, equally imbalancing, over-activity of the immune centers (autoimmunity) makes us susceptible to any and every type of illness. A few red flags telling you your immunity is out of whack include fatigue (cardiovascular and nervous centers), poor wound healing (all six centers), diarrhea (digestive center), allergies (respiratory center), and cancer (any of the six centers).

And what does your good, bad, or indifferent diet have to do with the high, low, or just fair functioning of each of these six centers that determine your well-being? Plenty. Read on.

Center One: Cardiovascular Center

This center includes the heart (no bigger than a clenched fist, it beats 3 million times a year), blood and blood vessels (60,000 miles of them), and the circulatory system. Blood moves from the heart to the lungs, mixes with oxygen, and then circulates along with nutrients (e.g., those anthocyanins from your blueberry breakfast, that fiber from your lunchtime wrap) to wherever it's needed. What goes around comes around: that same oxygenated blood makes a return trip to pick up

Cardiovascular Center Conditions: Hypertension, heart attack, stroke, coronary artery disease, high cholesterol, angina, athero-sclerosis, congestive heart failure, arrhythmias, varicose veins, Raynaud's disease, and stress

Cardiovascular Center Super Immunity Foods: Oranges and other citrus fruits, flaxseed, onions and garlic, tomatoes, olives and olive oil, sea vegetables, tea

and dispose of toxins in your system. The blood vessels or arteries (which could circle the globe two and a half times if strung together) connect with smaller capillaries and veins to bring blood back to the heart. It should all work like clockwork if the specialized immune cells in this center—the white blood cells that defend against invaders and the platelets that help the system self-repair—are up to steam.

Center Two: Nervous Center

The brain has a mind of its own, and indeed, this center comprising brain, spinal cord, and complex network of nerves is telecommunications and intelligent design in action. The central nervous system is central to tasting, seeing, thinking, hearing, dreaming, breathing, and feeling pain and pleasure. Thin threads of nerves called neurons are bundled together and carry information back and forth like wires gathered on a telephone pole. Sensory nerves send messages to the brain by way of the spinal cord, and motor nerves carry messages back from the brain to all the muscles and glands. When a neuron is stimulated by heat, cold, touch, or sound vibrations, it generates an electrical pulse that travels the length of the neuron and then is carried by chemicals to the next cell, hot-potato style. Plenty of events from the outer and inner environments can interfere with this interplay—and plenty of foods can keep this center strong!

Nervous Center Conditions: Anxiety, depression, obsessive-compulsive disorder (OCD), attention deficit/hyperactivity disorder (ADHD), stroke, Alzheimer's disease (AD), multiple sclerosis (MS), Parkinson's, cerebral palsy, headaches and migraines, vision disorders

Nervous Center Super Immunity Foods: Berries, dark leafy greens, green foods, mushrooms, apples, potatoes, herbs and spices

Center Three: Glandular Center

The lymphatic system includes important organs: the spleen, thymus, tonsils, and lymph nodes, which continuously cleanse the body at the cellular level, eliminating toxins and debris and destroying depleted cells. Lymph nodes (carrying T and B cells) that fight infections are located in the neck, armpits, chest, pelvis, and groin.

> **Glandular Center Conditions:** Hypothyroid and hyperthyroid disorders, adrenal disorders, obesity, breast cancer, prostate cancer, various cancers, osteoporosis, infertility, diabetes, infections (viral and bacterial)
>
> **Glandular Center Super Immunity Foods:** Carrots, citrus fruits, green foods, sea vegetables, nuts and seeds, apples

Center Four: Digestive/ Detoxification Center

Think before you munch. Digestion begins in the mouth with the salivary glands and wraps up in the small intestine. But it is a long, complex journey. Immune cells in the mucosa of the digestive tract in the mouth, esophagus, stomach, small and large intestines, and gallbladder must all be well fed and functioning to keep you protected. The liver and pancreas are also digestive organs, as is the gallbladder. Even the nervous and circulatory systems interact with this immune center. Most digested molecules of food, for example, are absorbed through the small intestine. The viability of the specific cells involved in this process is essential to the next step: passage into the bloodstream and distribution to the rest of the body for storage or further chemical transformation.

The many steps in the digestion of carbohydrates, fats, protein, vitamins, water, and salts depend on how well immune cells in the eight organs of this system are working. The well-being of the immune cells in turn ensures that the hormones controlling digestion from the mouth to the pancreas and the hormones stimulating and inhibiting the appetite are in good working order.

In the liver, Phase I and Phase II enzymes defend the body against toxins. These two enzyme systems are central to your body's ability to defend itself against bacteria, viruses, parasites, and toxic chemicals. Because of the wide variety of chemical reactions these enzymes undertake, they are major players in the fight against disease and illness. Nutrition has a significant role in the activation of these enzymes, says Dr. Paul Talalay, John Jacob Abel Distinguished Service Professor of Pharmacology and Director of the Laboratory for Molecular Sciences at Johns Hopkins University School of Medicine in Baltimore. According to Dr. Talalay, when Phase I enzymes are activated, they seek out toxic substances to make them water soluble and easier to usher out of the body. When Phase II enzymes are activated, they detoxify the toxins produced by Phase I enzymes, render them inert, and remove them from the body. Highly reactive molecules called free radicals are sometimes produced by this drama and can be tamed by antioxidants in your system. Many foods can tamp down oxidative damage, including cruciferous vegetables such as broccoli and cauliflower, as well as foods high in antioxidant vitamins A and C.

Digestive Center Conditions: Acid indigestion, heartburn and gastroesophageal reflux disease (GERD), halitosis, irritable bowel syndrome (IBS), colitis, Crohn's disease, diarrhea, constipation, ulcers, hepatitis, diverticulitis and diverticulosis
Digestive Center Super Immunity Foods: Tomatoes, broccoli, nuts and seeds, yogurt, berries, squash, apples

Center Five: Musculoskeletal Center

The body has 206 bones, including the skull, which protects the brain; the spinal column, which protects the spinal cord; the ribs, which protect the heart, lungs, liver, and spleen; and the pelvis, which protects the bladder, intestines, and (in women) the reproductive organs. In addition, joints make the skeleton flexible. Bones contain three types of cells: osteoblasts, which make new bone and repair old; osteoclasts, which break down, sculpt, and shape bone; and osteocytes, which carry nutrients to and waste products away from bones. To both store and release nutrients into the bloodstream, strong bones need calcium, sodium, phosphorus, vitamin D, collagen, and dozens of trace minerals and phytonutrients. The musculoskeletal center also includes bone marrow, in which stem cells produce red blood cells and platelets to help with clotting and wound healing and to carry much-needed oxygen to the body's tissues.

This center also includes 650 muscles (which account for about half of your weight) that are connected to bones by tendons. All of your voluntary muscle movements are coordinated and controlled by the cerebral cortex and cerebellum in the brain and nervous system, while the involuntary muscles are controlled by structures in the brain stem.

Plenty of things big and small can go wrong with this center when diet and lifestyle go awry. But you can do plenty of things big and small to keep your bones and muscles immune from harm.

Musculoskeletal Center Conditions: Osteoporosis, osteopenia, osteoarthritis, rheumatoid arthritis, temporomandibular joint (TMJ) and dental disorders, MS, scoliosis, tendonitis
Musculoskeletal Center Super Immunity Foods: Broccoli, carrots, dark leafy greens, oats, whole grains, yogurt, sea vegetables, soy foods, apples

Center Six: Respiratory Center

....

Without oxygen, you would expire. We are all here because our respiratory centers are in good, if not excellent, working condition. The air that we breathe with the help of the diaphragm and other muscles in the chest and abdomen circulates via the blood to all parts of the body. We breathe in some twenty times a minute, inhaling air that passes through the nasal passages; is filtered, heated, and moistened; and then is sent to the back of the throat. That breath has a long journey to the lungs through the windpipe, past the vocal cords, and to the juncture of the ribs at the center of the chest.

Inside each lung are bronchial tubes, which branch into even smaller tubes, which end in millions (i.e., 300 million) of alveoli. The air in these alveoli sacs is so extensive that the filled sacs, if laid out flat, would cover an area one-third the size of a tennis court. These sacs bring in new oxygen and exchange it for waste products like carbon dioxide. The red blood cells help exchange old carbon dioxide for new oxygen and carry the fresh oxygen to all the cells throughout the body. Carbon dioxide meanwhile travels through the lungs, back up the windpipe, and out of the body. This amazing process works best if all the players are equipped—through super immunity nutrition—to do their job effectively and keep you oxygenated.

Respiratory Center Conditions: Asthma, allergies, bronchitis, colds, flu, pneumonia, emphysema, chronic obstructive pulmonary disease (COPD)
Respiratory Center Super Immunity Foods: Carrots, tomatoes, squash, herbs and spices, mushrooms, tea

From apples to zucchini, the next chapter covers all you need to know to transform your diet for super immunity—one food at a time.

IMMUNITY BOOSTERS

The Top Twenty-Five Super Immunity Foods

Now that you've met the body's six immune centers, meet the twenty-five foods that feed them best to keep your immunity at full throttle. Food, not pharmaceuticals, is still your best medicine. Indeed, yesterday's little black bag is today's big brown grocery bag filled with apples, oranges, peas, and the twenty-two other foods that have been selected for their powerful blend of immunity-boosting vitamins, minerals, antioxidants, and phytonutrients. After learning about each immunity-boosting food, discover the immunity-busting conditions (Chapter 3) and then try the easy recipes and menus in Chapter 4, and you may fend off your next cold or flu, keep migraines and fatigue at bay, or even help prevent one or more of today's major diseases such as cancer, heart disease, or diabetes.

Apples

....

SUPER IMMUNITY CENTERS

Apples benefit the cardiovascular, glandular, and digestive/detoxi-
fication immune centers.

A symbol of fertility, temptation, and immortality, the apple appears
in many religious traditions as a forbidden fruit. But nutritionally it
is prescriptive not forbidden. The *Malus domestica*, a member of the
rose family, was born in Central Asia and is now the most cultivated
tree fruit in the world. Today there are 2,500 varieties of the domes-
tic apple's wild ancestors grown experimentally, although few reach
us. The ones that do—from the crisp Gala, to the aromatic Braeburn,
to the tart Granny Smith, to the old-fashioned Winesap—provide
plenty of variety. Farther afield, at farmers' markets and through family farms, there are hundreds more unusual heirloom apples for sale.
(See Resources for more information.)

Super Immunity Strengths

According to folklore, the male larynx is called an Adam's apple
because it resulted when the forbidden fruit got stuck in Adam's
throat. And what better fruit to stick in your craw: apples should be
the apple of your eye if you're working on nutritional self-defense,
and they probably are if you're the typical McIntosh-eating American.
Individually, we each eat twenty pounds of *Malus domesticus* apiece
each year—that's roughly one Delicious, Ida Red, or Granny Smith
(or other variety) every four days. Paltry compared to the European
average of almost two a day, but a munch in the right direction.

Big McIntosh—Big Medicine. Apples supply dozens of phytochemicals, including the ocular and antiallergy flavonoid quercetin, and
more potassium than fresh oranges. Eating an apple a day is the same
as taking a megadose of natural vitamin C in terms of antioxidants and

flavonoids. Apples rank sixteenth on the U.S. Department of Agriculture's Oxygen Radical Absorbance Capacity (ORAC) values chart, a ranking that reflects a fruit's antioxidant density—or the food's capacity to destroy or subdue free radicals and block oxidative damage to cells. Apples are even more "fruitful" if you eat the peel, which contains triterpenoids—compounds that have anticancer activity, according to Cornell University researchers. Triterpenoids appear to halt the growth of cancer cells, especially breast, colon, and liver. The flavonoids and phenols also inhibit other chronic diseases; flavonoids like quercetin are also responsible for raising neurotransmitters and protecting the brain against Alzheimer's and dementia.

Apples even strengthen the gallbladder. These juicy fruit foods help you satisfy your daily requirement for water. One medium apple is 84 percent water and supplies almost 4 ounces of water. Better yet, apples are "negative calorie" foods (along with watermelon, berries, and zucchini). This means that at 80 calories per average fruit, they burn more calories than they add and provide a lot of don't-need-a-second-helping satiety.

A Top Fruit Food for Fiber. Every part of any apple is good medicine. Apples rank as one of the top fifteen fruits and vegetables, providing four kinds of fiber. The fiber called pectin in apples helps the body's hormone disposal system work more efficiently, stabilizing blood pressure. Apples cleanse and rejuvenate the intestinal tract (for super cleansing, juice your apple with some parsley) and provide 3 grams of fiber (as much as a slice of whole-grain bread) to help prevent constipation and encourage a healthy bowel environment.

Buying, Storing, and Preparing

▶ The only downside of an apple a day? If it's not organic, it could be lowering, not raising, your immunity—so buy organic whenever possible.

▶ Apples are characterized (along with apricots, nectarines, and pears) as climacteric fruits, which ripen on their own, although they don't become sweeter in the process.

▶ Refrigerate apples to shut off flavor production in the skin. Letting the fruit sit at room temperature before eating will reactivate skin aromatics. Most apples will keep two weeks refrigerated. (Fujis and Granny Smiths have a longer life.)

▶ Buy with purpose in mind. Rome apples are best for baking and applesauce, Jonagolds and Ida Reds are best for pies, and all-purpose reds include Cortland and the McIntosh.

▶ If sliced or cut apples have to wait to be served, squirt them with lemon or other citrus juice to retard oxidation and browning.

▶ Go to the source. Visit a local orchard in harvesting time and pick your own. (This makes for a fun family outing, so take the kids!)

Berries

SUPER IMMUNITY CENTERS

Berries benefit the cardiovascular, nervous, glandular, and digestive/detoxification immune centers.

"Doubtless God could have made a better berry," observed William Butler about the strawberry in the seventeenth century, "but doubtless he never did." But he has given us a lot to choose from when the strawberries run out.

What do berries, the quintessential fruit of summer, bring to the summer, winter, fall, or spring table and to our overall immunity? Nearly everything, since blueberries, cranberries, raspberries, blackberries, and strawberries are among the top twenty foods with the most antioxidants (wild blueberries top the list).

Super Immunity Strengths

Fruits contain flavonoids, and the more the flavonoids, the sharper your brain. Also, anthocyanins—phytochemicals that give fruits and flowers their vibrant colors—are the top-gun nutrients in berries.

Berry Benefits. Berries, especially blueberries, have manganese to keep bones strong and vitamin C to strengthen all six immune centers. And the list goes on. Thanks to their ellagic acid plus vitamin C content, cranberries, raspberries, and strawberries all suppress the growth of several cancers and provide cardiovascular protection. Eating more berries can reduce your risk of arthritis, specifically of the knee (where arthritis is most common), thanks to increased vitamin C. In a ten-year study by Yuanyuan Wang, Ph.D., of Monash University in Australia, those with higher intake of fruit had the lowest arthritis risk.

And don't worry about the caloric damage. Most berries, eaten fresh, deliver between only 50 and 70 calories per cup along with moderate amounts of fiber. What to reach for? Eat raspberries for the most fiber, blueberries for the highest antioxidant content, strawberries for the most vitamin C and fewest calories, and currants and blackberries for the most potassium, a nutrient essential in preventing stroke, high blood pressure, and osteoporosis. Read on for more specific benefits of different berries, and pile them all on your plate for a super immunity defense.

Boost Night Vision with Bilberries. Bilberries (also called European bilberries) are at the top of the list, enhancing microcirculation in the capillaries, which in turn strengthens the retina, improving everything from macular degeneration to glaucoma, night vision, and cataracts. The therapeutic dose to affect change in the visual field is between 400 and 2,000 milligrams daily of standardized bilberry extract. (It takes 100 pounds of bilberries to extract 1 pound of extract.) After bilberries come blueberries, their American cousin.

Blueberries for Eyes, Allergies, and Cognitive Health. During the Civil War, soldiers drank blueberry juice to ward off scurvy. We still drink it for the vitamin C and a whole lot more. Blueberries protect your eyes from the damaging effects of sunlight, prevent and treat allergies, and also help with varicose veins.

Blueberries are also known as "the brain berry" because studies by James Joseph at the USDA's Human Nutrition Research Center on

Aging have shown that daily consumption of blueberries dramatically slows age-related impairment in memory and motor coordination. Blueberries also help lower cholesterol, promote urinary tract health, halt cataract progression, and protect against glaucoma.

And it's not just the berry itself. Blueberry leaf tea helps people with diabetes to rid the blood of excessive sugar, is useful in treating diarrhea, and keeps the kidneys healthy.

Take a Strawberry Shortcut Against Arthritis. Strawberries, perhaps our favorite summertime berry, are grown in twenty different varieties and are a good low-calorie (45 per cup) source of quercetin, another flavonoid that fights free radicals. The anthocyanins in strawberries are mild cyclooxygenase (COX) enzyme inhibitors, protecting against inflammatory conditions such as arthritis and general oxidative damage to cells.

EMS for UTIs. When it's the season for it, reach for the fresh cranberries, which fight urinary tract infections (UTIs) by preventing harmful bacteria such as *E. coli* from adhering to bladder walls and *H. pylori* bacteria from causing ulcers, according to Rutgers University researchers. The anthocyanins in cranberries (as in oranges, which cranberries partner well with) also help normalize cholesterol and improve blood circulation. Blueberries provide the same benefits.

Blackberries for Your Health. Ripe blackberries are life-giving, from the seeds to the leaves (which, like blueberry leaves, can be brewed as a healing tea). Due to their ellagic acid, blackberries are useful in reversing constipation, diarrhea, anemia, and cancer. They supply beta-carotene, iron, potassium, calcium, and even tocotrienols, which help inhibit cholesterol production in the liver. Blackberries have more fiber (8 grams per cup) than four pieces of whole wheat toast. Blackberries are one of the six best sources of folate, which helps convert homocysteine, a risk factor for heart disease, into methionine, a powerful antioxidant and chelating agent. Berries are also an important source of vitamin C, which helps produce the collagen important to bone, joint, and connective tissue health.

Exotic Berries, Exceptional Benefits. Or think outside the bowl and treat yourself to the exotic acai berry from Brazil's northern Amazon or the goji berry from Tibet. With an ORAC value that's higher than any other berry grown, the acai has twice the amount of antioxidants of blueberries, ten times that of grapes and cranberries, and thirty times the anthocyanins of red wine. The acai has plant sterols to reduce cholesterol, has antibacterial properties, and is used to improve circulation and sex drive as well.

But, says the Department of Plant Biology at the University of Illinois at Urbana-Champaign, the combined effect of the compounds working together is what makes them powerful medicine. Similarly, the slightly sweet-and-sour goji berry, usually sold dried, is rich in a cross section of antioxidants, especially the carotenoids, and has been used for promoting longevity, protecting the eyesight, protecting the liver, and, of course, improving immunity.

Buying, Storing, and Preparing

▶ For biggest flavor and smallest environmental impact or carbon footprint, buy berries locally and buy in season.

▶ Open the container of fresh berries, and immediately discard any overripe ones to prevent spoilage. Spread on a shallow plate, cover with paper towels, and refrigerate.

▶ Buy organic to avoid pesticides and herbicides. Berries (like peaches) are difficult to grow organically since 20 to 30 percent of the crop is lost to disease, defects, and predators, but the extra price is worth it. Whatever you buy, wash well using a vegetable and fruit wash, water spiked with hydrogen peroxide (1 tablespoon to each quart of water), or a vinegar-salt mixture (2 tablespoons of white vinegar and 1 teaspoon of salt to each quart of water).

▶ Fresh and frozen blueberries have more anthocyanins than dried.

▶ Don't rinse fresh berries until you're ready to use them, since rinsing encourages rot.

▶ Fresh cranberries can be frozen unwashed in their store-bought containers for up to one year. For other berries, wash (except for blueberries) and drain, place on a cookie sheet, and freeze. Then transfer them to a freezer bag. They keep up to twelve months.

▶ Buy frozen if fresh are unavailable. They are just as nutritious frozen, but not so if canned.

▶ Refrigerate most berries, and use within the week (ten days for blueberries).

▶ Avoid canned cranberry sauce, which has three times the calories of fresh berries and 86 percent less vitamin C.

Broccoli and Broccoli-Family Vegetables

SUPER IMMUNITY CENTER

Broccoli benefits the cardiovascular, nervous, glandular, digestive/detoxification, musculoskeletal, and respiratory immune centers.

Why add a stalk of broccoli to your super immunity diet? Think sulforaphane (an anticancer compound that's just one nutritional benefit of broccoli) when you think super immunity. Think bump in immunity when you put that forkful of broccoli, kale, or collards in your mouth.

Super Immunity Strengths

In addition to sulforaphane, that plate of cauliflower or handful of broccoli sprouts gives you another chemo-protective phytochemical, indole-3-carbinol (I3C), which helps normalize hormone balance and support liver detoxification. And eat up if you're getting on in years. Broccoli and broccoli family vegetables slow down the growth of cataracts, a common condition among the over-sixty-five population.

All of the broccoli plant is edible. Broccoli leaves, though rarely eaten, are even more nutritious than the stems and florets. Best of all, that's not all. Broccoli can double as one glass of water. With 91 percent water, each half cup of the plant provides 2.7 ounces of water (almost twice the water in a half cup of lettuce). That dish of stir-fried brussels sprouts, stuffed cabbage, or kale soup can also protect you from the common cold and seasonal allergies. The entire brassica family of vegetables—spinach, cauliflower, cabbage (from savoy to bok choy), collard greens, kale, and kohlrabi dish up the same benefits. Read on for more super immunity broccoli benefits.

Slow Aging, Lower Cholesterol, Fight Free Radicals. According to researchers at Johns Hopkins University School of Medicine, the compound sulforaphane, found in broccoli, broccoli sprouts, cauliflower, cabbage, and other brassica family vegetables, stimulates the antioxidant genes and enzymes and weakens the effects of free radicals that cause the oxidative damage that sets the stage for killer diseases such as cancer. Sulforaphane even slows down age-related decline in immune function and helps stabilize cholesterol levels. What's true for broccoli is especially true for broccoli sprouts, which contain 10 to 100 times more sulforaphane than mature broccoli.

Beat Ulcers, Eat More Kale. Sulforaphane has been effective against the *H. pylori* bacteria, one of the world's commonest bad bacteria, credited with causing 90 percent of intestinal ulcers and 80 percent of all stomach ulcers, according to the Centers for Disease Control and Prevention (CDC).

Broccoli for Bones. Broccoli can be your glass of milk. One cup supplies 41 milligrams of calcium for a healthy menstrual cycle and normal blood pressure, besides bone density. Plus that 1 cup includes vitamin C to encourage absorption of that calcium and vitamin K, which is also needed for skeletal health, minus the calories and saturated fat of dairy.

Multivitamin in a Stalk. Broccoli is abundant in vitamins C, K, and A (before you slice and dice, know that there is eight times more vitamin A in the raw florets than in the stalks) and chock-full of folate and dietary fiber, as well as B vitamins, protein, and even some omega-3 fatty acids. In fact, broccoli gives you 142 percent of what the government considers your daily value (DV) for vitamin C (75 mg), and since twenty-five times that value is safe, have seconds.

Brassica vegetables, says the Center for Science in the Public Interest, rank among the top ten healthiest vegetables, giving you the most vitamin C, folate, potassium, calcium, iron, carotenoids, and fiber. Kale and spinach rank at the top of vegetables with the highest ORAC scores.

In Taoist terms, broccoli has a neutral essence and enters the heart and large intestine meridian, energetically speaking. It benefits the heart and liver, according to traditional Chinese medicine, as it impacts the body's internal chi. (By contrast, cauliflower increases kidney energy, heals constipation, and benefits the gallbladder.)

Buying, Storing, and Preparing

▶ Pay the extra buck (or less) and buy organic. According to the USDA, levels of calcium in conventionally grown broccoli measured between 1973 and 1997 have dropped by 53 percent and riboflavin by 48 percent because of the denatured state of soil subjected to synthetic fertilizers, pesticides, herbicides, and irrigation practices.
▶ Never microwave your cruciferous vegetables, including broccoli. According to a 2006 report in the *Journal of the Science of Food and Agriculture,* zapping broccoli caused a 97 percent loss of nutrients. Steaming (5 minutes or less) trumps all other cooking methods.

▶ According to an American Chemical Society report, vegetables such as broccoli, carrots, and zucchini reserve or even boost their antioxidant power when cooked. Best way to fix cauliflower? Cook florets in vegetable broth for 5 minutes.

▶ Store broccoli stalks in a glass of water in the fridge to keep them from drooping (this works with asparagus, too).

▶ Broccoli sprouts are here today, gone tomorrow. To discourage spoilage, keep them in the original container. Use up within seven days.

▶ Eat your broccoli (and other cruciferous vegetables) both raw and cooked. It's richer in vitamin C when raw but higher in carotenoids when prepared.

Carrots

> **SUPER IMMUNITY CENTERS**
>
> Carrots benefit the cardiovascular, glandular, and digestive/detox-ification immune centers.

Carrot in front of your nose? Get it in your mouth, and your eyes will thank you. So will almost everything else below your line of vision.

Super Immunity Strengths

If there aren't carrots in your Monday-through-Sunday salads, lunch bags, soups, and juices, there should be. Here's why you need to get on the stick.

Beta-Carotene for Better Vision. Thanks to their high beta-carotene content, carrots do more for your vision than almost any other single vegetable. Make that now-and-then carrot a one-a-day carrot, and you lower your risk of macular degeneration, as well as improve your night vision.

Good for the Gut. Moving south, Bugs Bunny's comfort food is a comfort for your gastrointestinal tract and liver, too. Carrots contain complex sugars called oligosaccharides that prevent diarrhea by discouraging bad bacteria from attaching to the intestinal wall. The Physicians Committee for Responsible Medicine (PCRM) recommends carrots for colitis and other intestinal disorders. And like beets and burdock, carrots are a good, safe, liver-cleansing, and detoxification food.

Heart Health. And your heart isn't far behind. The high-fiber content in carrots reduces LDL cholesterol and raises good HDL cholesterol, and the combination of fiber and carbohydrates boosts serotonin levels and creates a feeling of relaxation.

Anticancer Crunch. Your lungs will thank you, too, for opting for carrot juice instead of a cola. Studies show that eating one medium-sized raw carrot four times a week reduces your risk of lung cancer. Carrots even reduce your colon cancer risk, thanks to the phytochemical falcarinol.

Bone Boost. The vitamin K in carrots helps build bone (especially when paired with a dark K-rich green like chard).

Buying, Storing, and Preparing

- ▶ Look for deep red-orange—a signifier that the carrots are high in beta-carotene.
- ▶ Choose medium sized and slender, not big, which tend to be fibrous and tough.
- ▶ Go for crisp, not limp, carrots.
- ▶ Carrots beg to be juiced, and you should oblige. They combine well with parsley, beets, and dark leafy greens, and, of course, garlic.

▶ Cooked carrots give you more antioxidants than do raw carrots. Steaming for 5 minutes produces the most vitamin A and beta-carotene.

▶ Place raw washed carrots in a storage bag and refrigerate.

Citrus Fruits

. . . .

> **SUPER IMMUNITY STRENGTHS**
>
> Citrus fruits benefit the cardiovascular, glandular, digestive/detox-ification, and musculoskeletal immune centers.

On an average day, 50 percent of all Americans eat no fruit at all, according to the USDA. But when they do, they (and perhaps you, too) are likely to reach for an orange. Citrus are surpassed only by apples and bananas in terms of the quantity in which they are pro-duced and eaten—and they're a good choice. Besides helping pre-vent your next rhinovirus infection, the flavones in oranges reduce LDL (bad) cholesterol and increase the good HDL. All our favor-ite citrus—from street oranges to exotic satsumas—are also rich in vitamin C, folate, potassium, and bone-building vitamin D, as well as capillary-supporting and antiviral bioflavonoids. But that's not all.

Super Immunity Benefits

An orange a day provides big nutritional self-defense for four of the body's immune centers—starting with digestion-maximizing and cholesterol-minimizing fiber.

Easily Digested Fiber. That grapefruit or tangerine beats bacon at breakfast. Unlike meat, which has no fiber and creates waste products during the forty-eight-hour digestion period, high-fiber, fat-free citrus is efficiently digested two hours after you put your grapefruit spoon away, advises Elson Haas, M.D., at the Preventive Medical Center of Marin in California, making citrus a perfect immunity-boosting breakfast starter.

Drink OJ for LDL. According to researchers at the Hebrew University of Jerusalem, the flavones in oranges stabilize cholesterol levels so effectively that high cholesterol sufferers might consider upping their intake of oranges before downing statin meds. (But remember, statin meds and most other prescription drugs don't mix with grapefruit juice, which increases the effects of many meds.) Citrus fruits like grapefruit also provide pectin, a soluble fiber that helps regulate cholesterol.

Think Citrus, Think Cancer-Fighting. Like tomatoes, red (but not white) grapefruit supplies lycopene, one of the top ten nutrients for fighting off and preventing prostate cancer and heart disease. A grapefruit supplies more lycopene than do sun-dried tomatoes or sweet red peppers.

According a recent Nurses' Health Study, women with the highest intake of luteolin, a flavone found in oranges and other citrus (as well as spinach and broccoli) had a 34 percent reduction in ovarian cancer risk, the fourth leading cause of cancer death among women.

Ascorbic Acid, Plus. Citrus fruit offers four times the vitamin C of bananas and more than three times the ascorbic acid of apples. If it's organic, you get 30 percent more vitamin C, according to researchers at Truman State University, plus a healthy dose of potassium. Potassium helps lower blood pressure and risk of stroke and is in short supply in the traditional diet. If you're getting your share (2,700 mg to 3,500 mg), you're probably eating oranges or drinking orange juice, which rank above bananas as a source.

Boosts Iron Absorption. The ascorbic acid in citrus boosts your body's absorption of non-heme iron found in plants. Having a glass of grapefruit juice before you fork up that spinach salad can help you absorb two to four times as much energizing iron as that salad would supply solo, according to the American Heart Association. The vitamin C in that lemonade or grapefruit also boosts your production of collagen for healthy, youthful-looking skin.

Citrus for Your Cerebellum. All citrus contain flavonoids for stronger brain power and a sharper mind. Try a cup of grapefruit sections raw at breakfast sprinkled with soy lecithin granules (for more cerebral muscle) or toss tangerine sections or a few kumquats in your tossed salad at lunch. Do citrus, not Xanax. Up your mood by squeezing a lemon wedge into a glass of water. According to Japanese scientists, the scent of lemon affects a portion of the brain called the cerebellum, lifting your spirit and reducing mental fatigue. A whiff of lemon is also said to affect stamina.

Fruit or Juice? A citrus juice like grapefruit juice, says a study by the University of Florida, contains more nutrients per calorie than apples, prunes, grape, or pineapple juices. Oranges have an ORAC rating of 750, surpassed by only eight other fruits. To limit both calories and sugars, choose the tangerine or navel orange over the juice. A glass of OJ adds 110 calories and 20 grams of sugar (as much as a small Almond Joy) to your daily totals. (A warning to people with diabetes: fruit juice raises blood sugar levels faster than a whole citrus does, because the high fiber of the fruit is digested more slowly.) High blood sugar levels make it harder to lose weight and may predispose you to type 2 diabetes. A third reason to reach for the whole fruit rather than the carton or can is that processed juices are heated and pasteurized, destroying some of the vitamins A, C, E, and B complex and, just as important, damaging the enzymes that aid in digestion and detoxification.

Sipping (Not Staring at) Our Navels: The Most Nutritious Fruit Juices. On the other hand, according to a report in *Pediatrics*, children who drink orange, pineapple, and other fruit juices have higher intakes of potassium, folate, and vitamin C. Oranges are citrus with the highest visibility. But there are plenty of other-than-oranges citrus worth bringing home. Consider other members of this large extended family:

- ▶ Blood orange (including Ruby Red, Moro, and Tarocco)
- ▶ Mandarin oranges (satsumas and clementines)
- ▶ Tangelos (a cross between the mandarin and the grapefruit)
- ▶ Ugli fruit (outsized tangelos from Jamaica)
- ▶ Murcott (a cross between the tangerine and the sweet orange)
- ▶ Grapefruit (white, pink, red, and golden)
- ▶ Pomelo (Chinese grapefruit)
- ▶ Lemons (including Eureka, Lisbon, and Meyer)
- ▶ Limes (including Persian, Kaffir, and Mandarin)
- ▶ Kumquat, almost the only citrus with an edible skin (The Meyer lemon can be eaten whole but probably rarely is.)

There are even the sour tangerine-sized Japanese yuzu, the limequat, and the lemonquat among the oddball citrus.

Buying, Storing, and Preparing

- ▶ Eat locally grown citrus. Citrus fruits imported from other countries are invariably fumigated, and all the travel miles leave a big carbon footprint.
- ▶ Pick fruit that is ripe, small, thin-skinned, but heavy for its fruit. If organic, don't demand cosmetic perfection.
- ▶ Think twice about commercial oranges that may have been dyed red to appear ripe and waxed (thus trapping pesticide residues) for a longer shelf life. Nonorganic citrus is sprayed with fifty different pesticides, and traces always remain.
- ▶ Avoid green oranges. They're less sweet because they haven't matured, are lower in vitamin C, and may aggravate existing joint pain.
- ▶ Chill your citrus to keep it fresh, but bring it to room temperature before eating or cooking with it.
- ▶ Wash with a vegetable wash or rinse with hydrogen peroxide (one tablespoon to a quart of water) before eating to remove mold, bacteria, and pesticide residue (if commercial).

Dark Leafy Greens

SUPER IMMUNITY CENTERS

Dark leafy greens benefit nervous, digestive/detoxification, and musculoskeletal immune centers.

Turn over a new leaf—a dark green one like one of the following eight healthiest dark leafy greens: dandelion, arugula, kale, collard greens, spinach, beet greens, romaine lettuce, and red leaf lettuce.

Super Immunity Strengths

Dark greens such as collards and spinach—not to mention mustard and dandelion greens, Swiss chard, and kale—are among the top ten healthiest vegetables you can pile on your plate, according to the Center for Science in the Public Interest. Besides folate, potassium, calcium, iron, carotenoids, fiber, and vitamin C, greens bring to the plate ammunition to fight off anything that threatens to compromise your immunity, from your neurotransmitters to your Achilles' heel.

Have a Salad; You'll Be Smarter for It. According to the Chicago Health and Aging Project (CHAP), eating just three servings of green leafy, yellow, and cruciferous vegetables daily can slow mental decline by 40 percent—a mental boost equal to five years of younger age! Conversely, researchers at UCLA studying the diets of 500 seventy- to seventy-nine-year-olds found that those whose diets were lowest in folate-source foods like leafy greens showed a 60 percent greater risk of serious cognitive decline. If they had rounded off their three square meals with a dark leafy green like spinach or collard greens, they might have been winning at Scrabble and acing those crossword puzzles.

Use some of that frisée to replace some of the fries in your diet, and you could benefit even more. According to the National Cancer

Institute, reducing your fat intake by just 6 percent can equal a significant reduction in your chances of developing cancer. Two reasons? Dark, leafy vegetables like kale and arugula are a source of vitamin E and folate, both critical for the activity of neurotransmitters and for discouraging the activity of tumors, especially breast, stomach, and color cancer, according to the National Women's Health Resource Center.

Try These Super Immunity Greens

Chard. Chard (or Swiss chard) with golden-orange, green, or ruby stalks provides 15 percent of your daily value for magnesium, vitamin C, bone-building vitamin K, and beta-carotene. In less time than it takes to order those bad-for-you fries, you could have this good-for-you Chard Stir-Fry: Heat 1 teaspoon olive oil, and sauté ¼ cup chopped onions (any kind), a dash of garlic powder, and ½ teaspoon lemon juice. Add ¼ cup white wine and 4 large stalks of chopped chard (dice stalks finely). Stir until chard wilts. Sprinkle with kelp powder, crushed dulse, or salt, and top with grated dairy or nondairy cheese. (Optional: add flaxseeds or soy lecithin granules.)

Spinach. First cultivated in Persia, spinach, along with kale, ranks at the top of the list of vegetables with the highest ORAC value (antioxidant potential). Besides eating your greens for vitamin E and folate, you're also getting vitamin C, which is more potent when combined with the vitamin E (tocopherol) in spinach. Most greens, including spinach, are a rich source of tocopherol and its subgroups (alpha, beta, gamma, and delta), which can reduce levels of C-reactive protein (CRP), a risk factor for heart disease. To benefit more, toss those greens with other sources of vitamin E such as nuts and omega-3-rich oils like flax and walnut.

Baby spinach may be the best grown-up way to build bone, since it supplies almost 200 percent of your daily value for vitamin K, along with calcium and magnesium, three nutrients that interact to mineralize bone. A bargain at 7 calories per cup of raw leaves, spinach provides 20 percent of your daily requirement for beta-carotene, plus fiber, folate, and ascorbic acid. It's tasty raw, steamed, solo, or combined with other greens.

Dandelion Greens. Or how about passing up the spinach on your next shopping outing and adding dandelion greens (when in season) to the basket? These classically bitter (think broccoli raab) spring greens provide as much calcium as cottage cheese, without the fat and for less than 40 calories a cupful. Plus, they have more vitamin A than most other greens and a third of your DV for ascorbic acid, along with iron and potassium. Try sautéing with oil and garlic or juicing with carrots. They pinch-hit for spinach or kale in almost any recipe. Also, dandelion greens have a tonic effect on the entire body, especially the liver and the gallbladder.

Lettuce. Let us eat our lettuce—and we certainly do: it's the second most popular vegetable in the United States. But let us choose wisely. Romaine has eight times the beta-carotene of iceberg lettuce and five times the vitamin C (as well as most other nutrients). There is another reason to pass on the iceberg: it takes 36 calories of fossil fuel just to grow and ship this low-nutrient green. And that's not all. Darker green lettuces like romaine and red leaf are superior to paler greens across the nutritional spectrum.

Cress. Take watercress (which is actually a member of the cabbage family). According to studies from the University of Ulster in Ireland, eating a large serving of watercress daily for eight weeks produced a 23 percent reduction in DNA damage to white blood cells and a 33 percent rise in beta-carotene and lutein in the body, safeguarding cells against cancer.

Chewing a few stems a day of this peppery green improves digestion and will help improve most illnesses, say naturopathic physicians, especially anemia, liver and thyroid problems, and arthritis. Chew watercress for its detoxifying properties if you are exposed to secondhand smoke. It's also an excellent green to add to the mix when you are juicing carrots, celery, and cucumber. If you must toss up an iceberg salad, this is an excellent green for added taste and nutritional punch.

Buying, Storing, and Preparing

▶ Spinach is tastiest from March to May and from September to October. As one of the twelve foods flagged by the Environmental Working Group for high levels of pesticide residue, be safe and buy organic.
▶ Spinach is one of the three vegetables (along with Swiss chard and beet greens) that are best boiled. Boiling releases oxalic acid, the substance that makes food taste bitter and may interfere with the body's ability to absorb some nutrients.
▶ Store greens unwashed and wrapped in a dampened paper towel inside a plastic bag until ready to use. Wash well and dry in a salad spinner or with an absorbent towel.

Green Food Powders

SUPER IMMUNITY CENTERS

Green food powders benefit the glandular, digestive/detoxification, and musculoskeletal immune centers.

Dark green leafy vegetables are good, but green foods like cereal grasses, such as barley and wheatgrass, and blue-green algae (BGA), such as spirulina and chlorella, are a real step up from good. This is especially true if, like most people, you are half a squash and a tomato away from meeting that five-a-day vegetable quota.

Super Immunity Strengths

You can stir broccoli sprouts into your salad, sprinkle spirulina in your soup, and mix sea vegetables into your vegetable juice (V8), but if you still come up short or want to get extra nutritional credit, why not multitask a little less and get a lot more of everything by adding green food powders once or twice a day to yogurts, water, and dips?

Green foods come in nutritional powder concentrates that include cereal grasses, such as barley and wheat, and blue-green algae, such as spirulina and chlorella. This minimum mixture gives you protein, enzymes, beta-carotene, chlorophyll, and trace minerals. Depending on the brand of nutritional powder concentrate, you might get a whole lot more: dried vegetables, fruits, grains, herbs, and spices along with bee pollen and probiotics may be added to boost healing powers.

A spoonful of green food powders gives you the equivalent of 3½ pounds of fresh vegetables—sometimes as many as forty-four different vegetables—grains, herbs, and spices. Green food powders stimulate the cells, rejuvenate the entire body, build red blood cells, and promote fast energy, according to the Hippocrates Health Institute where wheat grass first became popular. Better yet, according to Jerry Hickey, R.Ph., Chairman of the Society of Natural Pharmacy, green foods tone the intestinal tract and support digestion, detoxify and support the liver, provide energy, and reverse cellular inflammation.

The BGA Benefits. Chlorella is a single-celled, waterborne green alga that delivers more chlorophyll than any other known plant, more vitamin B_{12} than liver (usually found only in animal foods), and high levels of the antiaging nucleic acids DNA and RNA. Chlorella also supplies plenty of energizing B vitamins, vitamins C and A, protein, enzymes, and trace minerals. Spirulina, another microalgae, is also rich in B_{12} (a boon for vegetarians), nucleic acids, iron, and three essential fatty acids (EFAs). Both BGAs are highly digestible and can be used during dieting or fasting to provide all the nutrition needed to cleanse and rehab your system while keeping the appetite under lockdown. Because both microalgae are high in protein, a little bit can go a long way to stabilize blood sugar between meals for people with hypoglycemia.

Super Blades of Grass. The juice of barley grass, the young grass of the barley plant, is used to treat gastrointestinal disorders, arthritis, hepatitis, ulcers, asthma, and more. Is it any wonder? Rich in vitamin B complex and beta-carotene, it also provides a form of vitamin E called alpha-tocopherol succinate, which helps regulate reproductive hormones and may be useful in suppressing tumors. Barley grass is rich in seven minerals, including the antioxidant enzyme superoxide dismutase (SOD), which destroys superoxide. The most common free radical in the body, superoxide increases with age, causing wrinkles and precancerous cell changes, according to the Linus Pauling Institute.

Mow the Grass, Get Your Minerals. Wheatgrass, the young grass that sprouts when wheat kernels are planted, is nutritionally superior to all land-grown plants and supplies virtually all the minerals needed for super immunity. Wheatgrass uniquely works directly on the liver for healing and detoxification of heavy metals and other toxins, cleansing the blood and improving the health of the bowel without chemical stool softeners and laxatives. Wheatgrass is often sold as a living plant or as a juiced-on-the-spot additive to other fresh juices at juice bars and health food markets.

This nutrient-rich grass contains seventeen amino acids, which are the building blocks of proteins, essential for things like building muscle tissue, repairing cells, and clotting the blood. Wheatgrass retains 92 of the 102 minerals found in the soil, including calcium, phosphorus, iron, magnesium, and potassium. It is a rich natural source of vitamins A and C.

Richer than Carrots and Oranges. Wheatgrass has more vitamin C than oranges and twice the vitamin A of carrots. It is rich in vitamins E, K, and B complex, and a natural source of laetrile (vitamin B_{17}).

Figs and Dates

SUPER IMMUNITY CENTERS

Figs and dates benefit the digestive/detoxification, musculoskeletal, and respiratory immune centers.

The ancients attributed "magical powers" to figs, while the Egyptians treasured them for their digestive and cleansing properties and buried whole baskets of figs with their dead. Varieties include Weeping, Creeping, Wavy-Leaved, and Sacred figs. There are seventy species of *Ficus carica* in Asia alone. The ficus is one of the two sacred trees in Islam, and the Buddha sat under a ficus tree to find enlightenment. You have plenty of reasons to give a fig about figs. Nothing equals the taste (it's luscious) or the life span (it's short: they last just seven days from harvest to your mouth), and the *Ficus carica* is a clear-conscience way to satisfy a sweet tooth without reaching for a candy bar. There are 700 varieties of this tree, historically known as the "Tree of Life." Curiously, the fig is actually a flower, the seeds of which constitute the fruit.

Comprising 80 percent sugar, figs or dates especially make a great natural sugar or syrup substitute. But there's more.

Super Immunity Strengths

Figs and dates are rich in potassium and help stabilize cholesterol and blood pressure. Plus, the antioxidant phenols they supply protect against heart disease. Just three to four figs provide 100 milligrams of calcium for strong bones and a strong heart, plus the trace mineral manganese for healthy bones and wound healing. Dates also provide twenty different amino acids (the building blocks of protein, which control all cellular processes), along with bone-strengthening boron and magnesium. To boot, they have more potassium than bananas, plus beta-carotene for anticancer benefits. Fig leaves have super immunity benefits, too; they have an antidiabetic effect, lowering insulin as well as triglycerides, which are a risk factor for heart disease.

Buying, Storing, and Preparing

▶ Buy sulfur-free, dried fruits. Ten percent of all people with asthma are sensitive to the preservative sulphur dioxide, which offers no health benefits.
▶ Fresh figs should be soft but not mushy. Dates are smooth-skinned, glossy, and plump.

▶ Store ripe figs (the riper they are, the more antioxidants) in a shallow paper-towel-lined dish and refrigerate, covered with plastic wrap. Fresh figs can be ripened at room temperature. Dried figs keep for months tightly wrapped, stored in an airtight container in or out of the fridge.

▶ Wash figs and dates under cold water.

▶ For easier slicing, place figs and dates in the fridge for an hour; dip scissor blades in water before snipping either open.

Garlic

SUPER IMMUNITY CENTERS

Garlic benefits the cardiovascular, glandular, and digestive/detoxification immune centers.

According to folklore, when Satan left the Garden of Eden, garlic sprang up from his left footprint and onion from his right. From Satan's foot to our kitchen counters, garlic is full-body medicine. What it doesn't do for your arthritis, it does for your artheriosclerosis. If you don't have either, chances that you will dwindle with every spoonful of garlic soup and garlicky tomato sauce. Called the stinking rose, garlic is a member of the lily family, along with onions, chives, leeks, and shallots. Garlic was invoked as a deity by the ancients and enjoyed by the Romans but often reviled as a vulgar and even poisonous food in earlier Greco-Roman times. Born in Siberia, garlic traveled to Europe and became a staple in countries bordering the Mediterranean. Today it is grown and eaten for a variety of reasons (including improved immunity) worldwide.

Super Immunity Strengths

Garlic contains the plant fiber inulin, an insoluble fiber that helps lower cholesterol and blood glucose. Also found in chicory, onions, and leeks, inulin boosts good bacteria in the gut and improves absorption of both iron and calcium, according to plant physiologists at the USDA. Garlic also contains beta-carotene, zinc, selenium, and folate along with allicin, a chemical compound responsible for garlic's smell and bite, which is released only when garlic is crushed or cut.

There are some places garlic shouldn't go: it's contraindicated if you're on blood-thinning medication, for example. But for the rest of us fighting colds, heart disease, and worse, few foods are as immune-enhancing as *Allium sativum*. Garlic inhibits seventy-two distinct infectious agents, bacteria, fungi, and viruses, including those that cause the common cold, as well as candida and parasites. Garlic can protect you from the ulcer bacteria, *H. pylori*, and help detoxify heavy metals such as lead, cadmium, and mercury. There are ongoing studies on garlic's effect in reducing cancers of the stomach and the colon. A meta-analysis of studies at the University of North Carolina showed that eating ten cloves of garlic weekly reduced the risk of colon cancer by 30 percent and stomach cancer by 50 percent. Studies at New York University Medical Center in the 1980s showed that garlic oil could slow development of skin cancer.

Buying, Storing, and Preparing

▶ Garlic can thin the blood much like aspirin. Use conservatively if you are on a blood thinner, and check with your physician.

▶ The inulins in garlic can cause flatulence, especially if your diet is low in inulin-bearing foods. Start small and work your way up to larger amounts of garlic (and onion).

▶ Elephant garlic is actually not garlic but a wild leek used like garlic.

▶ Get your daily dose of allinase without an aftertaste. Cut one or two cloves into small slices, chew, and wash down with a glass of orange juice (for up to 30 percent more vitamin C, make it organic). This lets the garlic get immediately into your bloodstream, faster than with marinara sauce.

▶ Prepare it properly. Always crush the garlic and let it sit for a few minutes to allow the release of healing enzymes, per advice from scientists at the USDA. Never microwave garlic; this neutralizes its anticlotting effect. If using in cooking, add garlic near the end of the process.

► For the best flavor, look for hardneck garlic (as opposed to soft-neck), which has a strong inner stem.

► Choose bulbs that show no sprouting or loose skins.

► Store at room temperature to prevent sprouting, or buy in braided plaits and hang them in your kitchen.

Flaxseed

SUPER IMMUNITY STRENGTHS

Flaxseed benefits the cardiovascular, glandular, and musculoskel-etal immune centers.

Super Immunity Strengths

From thinner blood to tougher bones (and beyond,) flax is the seed to stock.

Flaxseed Builds Bone. Flaxseed is the number one source of alpha-linolenic acid (ALA), an omega-3 fat that is in short supply in the American diet. ALA is a precursor to the form of omega-3 fat in fish oil called eicosapentaenoic acid (EPA). The body converts ALA to EPA. If you want to truly supersize a meal, do something seedy—sprinkle or dribble in a little flaxseed or flaxseed oil. Plant-based fats like those in flaxseed help promote skeletal health by preventing excessive bone turnover.

Breast Cancer Protection. A report in the *European Journal of Cancer Prevention* noted that women with a higher flaxseed lignan (a compound with estrogenic and antioxidant properties) intake reduced their risk of breast cancer by 58 percent. Other studies show that thyroid cancer is lowest among those using flaxseed and soy in their diets. Duke University researchers report that flax helps slow the growth of prostate cancer by halting cellular growth. In the colon, omega-3 fats help protect colon cells from carcinogens and free radicals.

Cardiovascular Immunity. In studies conducted at Canada's University of Saskatchewan, secoisolariciresinol diglucoside (SDG), which is the primary lignan in flaxseed, decreased bad LDL cholesterol as well as total cholesterol and raised good HDL cholesterol. It also reduced the development of arteriosclerosis by 73 percent. People using flaxseed with the highest lignan levels also show the lowest increases in blood pressure under stress. (Read the labels, as these levels vary widely.) Flax also works as a mild blood thinner, inhibiting clots that could lead to stroke.

Anti-Inflammation. Flax prompts the body to increase production of anti-inflammatory prostaglandins along with magnesium to reduce the inflammatory process in joint disorders as well as asthma, allergies, osteoporosis, migraines, and psoriasis.

Disable Diabetes. Regular use of flaxseed lignans reduces the risk of diabetes by 75 percent, say University of Saskatchewan researchers. Also, the fiber in flaxseed helps stabilize blood sugar as well as protect the kidneys from the damage that often comes with this disorder.

Dry-Eye Relief. Reduce dry eye syndrome and conjunctivitis with docosahexaenoic acid (DHA), a natural component of flaxseed (also found in cold-water fish) that helps repair free-radical damage to retinal membranes; 300 to 500 milligrams a day does the trick.

Autoimmune Ammunition. Flaxseed is a potent source of omega-3 essential fatty acids (EFAs), which provide protection against autoimmune disorders such as Crohn's disease, irritable bowel syndrome, rheumatism, and inflammatory respiratory conditions.

Flax Lax. Flaxseed supplies 3 grams of fiber per ground tablespoon (as much fiber as a cup of raw carrots) to keep the intestinal tract healthy and prevent constipation. Use ground flax as a laxative in bran muffins, brew as a tea (pour 1 cup of boiling water over 2 tablespoons of flaxeed meal and steep for 10 minutes; strain and sweeten), or sprout flaxseed and use the sprouts on top of everything.

ALA for PMS. Plant-based fats such as the alpha-linolenic acid in flax can help alleviate menstrual symptoms. Sprinkle a little flaxseed on your morning cereal; dribble a little flaxseed oil on your tossed greens.

Five Flax Facts

- The name in Latin means "most useful": *Linum usitatissimum*.
- Flaxseed fibers can be woven into linen.
- Canada is the primary producer of flaxseeds.
- The health benefits of flaxseed were known in ancient Greece.
- The flax plant has been around since the Stone Age.

Buying, Storing, and Preparing

▶ What you take may not be what you get. For flaxseed's ALA fats to be converted to EPA, healthy levels of the enzyme delta-6 must be present. It is less available or less active in some of us, especially for people with diabetes or when eaten with alcohol and saturated fats. Take more flaxseed to get the same benefits you would with fish oils: three to four capsules of flaxseed oil for one fish oil capsule (or consult your health care professional). If you are a nonvegetarian, take both flax and fish oil supplements.

▶ Flaxseed is sold as a whole seed (the most potent), preground, as an oil, and in tablets, powders, and capsules. Use either the seeds or powder, plus the oil, to get the most lignans and fiber.

- ► Flaxseed is highly perishable. Don't buy more than you can use (bad oil is not good oil); be sure to refrigerate and use the oil up within three months.
- ► Use 1 to 2 tablespoons oil, seeds, or powder daily on salads, grains, and pasta. If you don't make your quota, take flaxseed oil capsules.
- ► Sprout whole flaxseeds. Flaxseed is mucilaginous and more challenging to sprout. So for best results, use a clay or bag sprouter (see Resources). Or mix the seeds with alfalfa and clover for a better harvest.

Legumes

SUPER IMMUNITY CENTERS

Legumes benefit the cardiovascular, glandular, and musculoskeletal immune centers.

"You can tell a lot about a fellow's character by his way of eating jellybeans," observed President Ronald Reagan. You can also tell a lot about a fellow just by the beans (hold the jelly) he adds or doesn't add to his diet. The more legumes you eat, the better. In fact, make it 3 cups a week, and you've got the upper hand on lowering cholesterol, stabilizing blood sugar, avoiding heart disease, and preventing diabetes, hypertension, obesity, and some cancers. With their high satiety value, providing bulk and fullness with few calories and fiber without fat, beans will also keep you fit.

This sprawling family includes everything from red clover, to mung beans, to peanuts, to even carob, the chocolate substitute. But best known are the dried beans such as chickpeas, kidney beans, black beans, and limas. Because of the high protein content beans offer, organizations such as the American Cancer Society recommend using beans as an alternative to meat. For example, 1 cup of lentils provides

17 grams of protein with one-sixth the fat (none of it saturated) of a lean steak. Note: except for soybeans, beans are not a complete protein. But they become a complete protein when you combine them with a grain such as brown rice or couscous either at the same meal or sometime during the same day.

Super Immunity Strengths

Use your bean and pick up your fork. Here are four big payoffs.

Osteo Answer. Have a grilled tofu burger in place of a cubed steak, and you avoid the acidity that in turn causes calcium loss from bones. That lean protein also comes with fiber, which is missing from meat, and phytonutrients, minerals, and vitamins.

Have a Heart: Eat a Bean Burger. In a nineteen-year study of almost 20,000 men and women, those who ate beans at least four times a week had a 22 percent lower risk of heart disease than those who had beans less than once a week. Keeping legumes on the menu also keeps blood pressure, triglycerides, and total cholesterol down (as efficiently as oat bran).

Insulin Resistance? Hypoglycemia? Diabetes? The fiber in that kidney bean chili or white bean soup keeps blood sugar levels from spiking and supplies a slow, steady stream of energy. Beans deliver 5 grams of fiber per serving (one-sixth of your daily DV for fiber), which qualifies those lentils, kidney beans, and peas as high-fiber foods.

Can Opener Against Cancer. Higher rates of bean consumption track with lower rates of cancer of the colon, breast, and prostate, according to epidemiological studies, thanks to the phytoestrogens called lignans, which appear to have a chemoprotective effect on tumors. Phytates, another phytochemical in beans, may be responsible for lower rates of intestinal cancer.

Buying, Storing, and Preparing

▶ Taste fresh (nondried) beans before you buy, to make sure of tenderness and sweetness before cooking.

▶ Make sure your dried beans are still fresh. Over-the-hill dried beans cook up tough.

▶ For gas-free beans, refrigerate or freeze extra cooking liquid from your first batch of beans and add it to your next batch when ready to cook. This infuses beans with gas-preventing bacteria.

▶ Cooking green beans? Keep the lid on. The riboflavin (vitamin B_2) they contain is light sensitive.

▶ Using canned beans? Look for organic and get low-sodium varieties. Rinse well to remove almost half of the salt.

▶ The longer you soak dried beans (preferably overnight), the shorter the cooking time.

Oats

SUPER IMMUNITY CENTERS

Oats benefit the cardiovascular, nervous, glandular, musculoskeletal, digestive/detoxification, and respiratory immune centers.

When you go "bowling" at breakfast, add oats. Used originally as medicinal food and originating in Asia as the red oat, oats have been cultivated for 2,000 years. The ancient Greeks were the first to eat oatmeal, which came to America in 1600 with the British immigrants-to-become-colonists. Oats support immunity; provide a stress-lowering amino acid (tryptophan) and a trace mineral for strong bones (manganese); and have more fiber for a healthy heart and colon than do blueberries or brown rice. Best of all, you can eat them in a cookie or a muffin. And why wouldn't you? *Avena sativa* (oats) in the bowl as cereal or in the hand as a cookie are a boon to all six immune centers.

Super Immunity Strengths

Oats lower total cholesterol, protect artery walls, protect against hypertension, improve immune response to infection anywhere in the body, stabilize blood sugar, and offer protection against breast cancer.

Lowering of Cholesterol Levels. Oats, oat bran, and oatmeal, which unlike other grains retain their fiber and nutrients even after hulling, supply a cholesterol-lowering fiber called beta-glucan. Consuming a bowl, or 3 grams worth, of this fiber daily lowers total cholesterol by 8 to 23 percent. Since a 1 percent drop in total cholesterol correlates with a 2 percent drop in the risk for developing heart disease, this is a breakfast choice that matters. Other studies have shown that eating 20 grams of fiber or more daily can produce a 12 to 15 percent drop in coronary and cardiovascular disease. Similarly, in the almost twenty-year-long Physicians' Health Study, participants who ate one bowl of whole-grain cereal (oat or another grain) showed a 29 percent lower risk for heart failure. Another blood lipid-lowering compound in oats, avenanthramides, prevents dangerous LDL cholesterol from oxidizing and becoming plaque on artery walls.

Protection from Blood Sugar Spikes. Beta-glucan fiber helps stabilize blood sugar in people with diabetes and improves insulin sensitivity by lowering glycemic content and hiking vitamin E, magnesium, and fiber content.

Buying, Storing, and Preparing

▶ Store oats in an airtight container in a cool, dry place (oats are slightly more perishable than other grains).
▶ Skip oats if you have celiac disease and must avoid gluten.

Olives and Olive Oil

....

Olives benefit the cardiovascular, nervous, and glandular immune centers.

If you haven't had your five servings of fruit today, reach for an *Olea europaea*. There's plenty to choose from: seventy-five major varieties of olives are cultivated worldwide. Botanically speaking, the olive is indeed a fruit in the same basket with apples, plums, and kiwis. Olives are among the world's oldest and least allergenic foods. Olive oil should be on your bread, your vegetables, your pizza, and in your refrigerator. It should not be on the countertop—at least not for long, as it perishes just like other fruits. Olives belong in your salads, bread spreads, and martinis (real or mock). Olives are a symbol of peace and wisdom, and what could be smarter than making olives and olive oil a part of your diet?

Did You Know That . . . ?
- There are 800 million olive trees on the earth today.
- Greece grows 93 percent of the world's olives.
- Annually, Greeks consume 6 gallons of olive oil per capita to the American 1 pint per capita.
- An olive tree can live for 600 years.

Super Immunity Strengths

Olives give you 25 percent of your iron, 20 percent of your vitamin E, and 17 percent of your fiber requirement. According to the National Institutes of Health, following a Mediterranean-style diet with plenty of olive oil makes you 20 percent less likely to die in the next five years. Olive oil protects the immune system, fends off weight gain, and reduces your chances of developing diabetes, heart disease, and cancer. An olive has only 18 calories, but it also gives you the amino acids leucine, aspartic acid, and glutamic acid; unsaturated fatty acids; vitamins E and A; and beta-carotene, as well as calcium and magnesium.

Fighting Four Disorders with Oleocanthal. Research from Philadelphia's Monell Chemical Senses Center have identified an anti-inflammatory agent similar to ibuprofen called oleocanthal in extra-virgin olive oil that reduces the inflammatory response that leads to dementia, heart disease, stroke, and breast cancer.

Buying, Storing, and Preparing

▶ Use oil labeled "olive oil" (actually a blend of olive and other oils) for cooking. It produces a crisp, rather than gummy, crust without greasiness. Use extra-virgin olive oil for salads and for dressing foods.

▶ Plastic containers can leak chemicals into the oil; buy olive oil only in glass and store it in a dark, dry place.

▶ To store olive oil, refrigerate all but expensive extra-virgin grades. Chilled oils may turn cloudy or solid, but that's not a red flag. Olive oil properly stored will keep up to two years.

▶ Olives should always be eaten at room temperature and stored in water, brine, or oil.

▶ Extra-virgin too pricey? Look for "combination" olive oils, which combine extra-virgin with everyday types.

Herbs and Spices

SUPER IMMUNITY CENTERS

Herbs and spices benefit the nervous, glandular, and respiratory immune centers.

As a source of good fun, humorist Dorothy Parker once remarked of an acquaintance, "She ranks somewhere between a sprig of parsley and a single ice skate." A single ice skate may be useless, but not so parsley (a name derived from the Greek for "rock celery"), which is perhaps the world's most celebrated herb.

Super Immunity Strengths: Herbs

Plenty of garden-variety herbs have better-than-garden-variety powers as immune boosters, and parsley is a good place to start stocking up.

Parsley Power. A cousin of the carrot and celery, curly leaf or flat leaf parsley has been used traditionally as a digestive aid, as a diuretic, to stimulate the kidneys, to improve the vigor of the lungs and spleen, and to freshen breath. Parsley also provides seventeen different vitamins and minerals, including 153 percent of your daily need for vitamin K for normal blood clotting. Every sprig supplies fiber for the heart and the colon, as well as a dozen phytochemicals that improve immunity throughout the body. Among them are chemoprotective volatile oils such as myristicin, which can neutralize carcinogens such as benzopyrenes found in charcoal and cigarette smoke. Parsley tea is drunk as a safe and effective diuretic. The flat-leaf variety provides both stronger flavor and slightly more nutrients. Store in a plastic bag and refrigerate.

Pesto Against Osteoarthritis. Or how about parsley's companion herb on the sill, basil? Once a symbol of love in Italy and of hospitality in India, basil is the anchor ingredient in pesto sauce. It contains the anti-inflammatory compound eugenol that blocks the activity of the COX enzymes in conditions such as osteoarthritis. Additionally, eugenol is an antibacterial shield against *Listeria*, *E. coli*, and many other bacteria. Basil is a superior source of vitamin K for strong bones as well as beta-carotene, magnesium, iron, calcium, and potassium. If you grow your own, you can choose from sixty different varieties, from sweet basil to cinnamon basil. Best way to dry for future use?

Dip whole leaves in boiling water and then soak in ice water. Pat dry and freeze in a single layer on a tray. Store in an airtight freezer bag.

Thyme and Rosemary: More than Seasoning. Like basil, thyme, one of the three herbs in the French bouquet garni, is an anti-inflammatory and antibacterial herb useful in healing respiratory conditions such as bronchitis. It is a good source of vitamin K and manganese for strong bones and healthy nerve function, as well as an insoluble plant fiber to control the pH in the intestines.

Rosemary is for remembrance but also much more. Rosemary has antibacterial properties and can be used to cleanse a room of negativity. A mild stimulant for the nervous system, it can be drunk to quell a headache. Used on the scalp, it prevents dandruff and encourages healthy hair and skin. Add a sprig of rosemary to a brewing pot of tea or lemonade. Use crushed leaves in any marinade.

Sleep Better, Smell Better with Mint. There are at least 3,500 varieties of this medicinal, therapeutic, and ornamental herb, of which the most popular are peppermint, which is the most effective therapeutically, and spearmint, which is the most favored for cooking. We keep them within reach for good reason. That cup of tea or saucer of mint sauce is just what the herbalist ordered for indigestion, flatulence, colic, a toothache, menstrual cramps, or even insomnia. Chewing on mint leaves will remedy bad breath, gargling with mint water or tea will ease a sore throat, and sniffing peppermint oil, say aromatherapists, stimulates the brain and improves productivity. Mint is hardy and easy to grow and comes back each year. Tired of mint? Step up to hyssop, a mint family member with edible blue flowers.

Super Immunity Strengths: Spices

Pepper, our most popular and bestselling spice, stimulates digestion, fights bacteria, and provides vitamins A and K as well as magnesium and potassium, but here are some other spices to keep the peppermill company.

Sweet Healing Cinnamon. No spice shelf is complete without cinnamon. Think sweet and pungent. Aromatherapists believe inhaling the scent of cinnamon spice improves mood, vigor, and concentration.

Curry Against Cancer. Turmeric (a root relative of ginger) is more than just the herb that gives curry its color. At the M. D. Anderson Cancer Treatment Center in Houston, Texas, curcumin extract (the healing compound in turmeric) is used as an adjunct to cancer therapy. That's not all: 2,000 studies have been published on the potent anti-inflammatory effects of turmeric and curcumin, which block inflammation through ninety-seven distinct mechanisms in the body, making it useful fight-back therapy for disorders caused by inflammation, such as heart disease, arthritis, irritable bowel syndrome (IBS), psoriasis, and ulcerative colitis. Try turmeric in pickles, pasta, and grain dishes; add it to soups, stews, and stir-frys. Sprinkle over open-faced sandwiches before broiling; stir into scrambled eggs or scrambled tofu dishes.

Boost Your Chi and Your Circulation with Ginger. Ginger is another go-to spice. The first gingerbread man found his legs 4,400 years ago in the Orient and he's still on the run. By the late 1800s, the British were importing 5 million pounds of it per year. According to traditional Chinese medicine, ginger has a warm essence, benefits the stomach, and keeps the liver chi flowing. A dose of this half-spicy, half-citrusy root relieves nausea, motion sickness, indigestion, and flatulence. A cup of ginger tea (double up, have a gingersnap too) will stimulate the circulation. Some studies indicate that ginger may help lower cholesterol and prevent blood clotting. Ginger can be eaten with onions and garlic as well as with rhubarb, peaches, fish, or anything else in your larder or fruit cellar. A refrigerated root (wrapped in a paper towel and stored in a plastic bag), which is more therapeutic than powder, will keep for up to one month. (To peel ginger, use the edge of a spoon. It gets into the corners and produces less mess.)

Mushrooms

....

Got *Agaricus bisporus* in your fridge or cupboard? It's a large family, so if you've only befriended the button, keep eating. You'll be in good fungi-friendly company. We Americans are buying and eating twice as many exotic mushrooms as we were ten years ago, according to the American Mushroom Institute. There's plenty of payback besides just taste. There are approximately thirty-eight species of edible mushroom in North America. None of them have more than 25 calories a half cup; all of them are low in sodium and have zero fat. Some of them are far tastier than others.

Super Immunity Strengths

The Egyptians considered the *Agaricus bisporus* a food fit for kings. Classical scholars have regarded mushrooms as the secret behind the Eleusinian Mysteries. In the Chinese culture, where mushrooms have been used as pharmaceuticals for centuries, they represent immortality and eccentricity (the latter because mushrooms are the only plant without leaves or flowers). There are exotic mushrooms like the portobello and the shiitake, and there are the mom-and-pop mushrooms like the button. All are rich in polysaccharides, the carbohydrate molecules that directly enhance the immune system and help lower the risk of breast cancer by inhibiting the circulation of estrogen. Mushrooms are also an excellent source of various B complex nutrients bound up with essential minerals such as potassium and selenium. Mushrooms, from the high-end shiitake to the humble button, all help lower blood pressure, fight cancer, and regulate immunity with every bite. Mushrooms also deliver a healthy dose of niacin, needed for healthy skin, healthy nerves, and good digestion.

Shiitake for Your Health. Also known as forest, Chinese dried, black, or flower mushrooms, shiitakes can be used dried or fresh. With their rich meaty flavor, they are (like the portobello) a valuable replacement for meat in meatless recipes. The most popular of the healing fungi, shiitakes have been used for centuries in Japan and China to treat colds and flu, poor circulation, upset stomachs, and exhaustion. They are also used as intervention for high blood pressure and heart disease, for lowering bad cholesterol, and for promoting longevity. Higher in both fiber and protein than button mushrooms, they are also useful in controlling *Candidiasis* (yeast infections). Their buttery flavor enhances broths, stir-fries, and sauces.

Mighty Maitake. Since feudal times, the crunchy, fragrant maitake mushroom has been used as a tonic to strengthen the body and improve overall immunity. Similarly, because it is classified as an adaptogen, a substance that helps the body adapt to stressors and restores equilibrium in the body, maitakes are your hot-ticket food for turning around a dozen disease states, from Lyme disease and chronic fatigue syndrome to cancer and Metabolic Syndrome X, a cluster of symptoms that put you at risk of diabetes and heart disease.

What Else Belongs in Your Mushroom Basket?

- Cremini are button fungi with an aggressive flavor rich in energizing riboflavin.
- Enokis have a sweet crisp texture and taste best raw. Use them as a garnish, crudités, or a substitute for sprouts. They are rich in vitamin D and the vitamin B complex.
- Portobellos are actually mature cremini mushrooms, rich in potassium and delicious grilled as a meat substitute.
- Porcinis are diminutive and earthy tasting with a woodsy aroma. Niacin and potassium are their star nutrients.

Buying, Storing, and Preparing

▶ Cooked mushrooms are more nutritious and a safer bet. Heat
makes their nutrients more available; in their raw state, mushrooms pass through your intestinal tract intact. Worse, some
types, including portobello, white button, and cremini, contain hydrazines, potentially carcinogenic compounds that are
destroyed by drying or cooking.

▶ Refrigerate in paper, not plastic. Once opened, mushrooms
should be stored outside the crisper drawer in an open paper bag
to prevent developing moisture.

▶ Choose whole, not sliced, mushrooms that are bright and not
bruised; they'll stay fresher longer. (But slightly discolored mushrooms are still nutrient-dense and can be eaten.)

▶ Spend the extra dollar for organic. Mushrooms grown in conventional soil can accumulate heavy metals and toxins, as well as
pesticides.

▶ Pass up conventional canned mushrooms. Processing leaches out
essential nutrients, and there is the possibility of contaminants
from both the soil and the canning process.

Potatoes

SUPER IMMUNITY CENTERS

Potatoes benefit the cardiovascular, nervous, and glandular
immune centers.

Potatoes have eyes; potatoes also have legs and they go the distance
for you nutritionally. They make good immunity-boosting medicine.
A potato or two, properly prepared, may even help keep your doctor
away. Potatoes are in fact the world's single most important vegetable,
grown in more countries (a hundred) than any other vegetable with

the exception of corn. We live on "a fry and a prayer" worldwide. We steam, broil, fry, sauté, shake and bake, roast, and pressure-cook, all in all, 100 billion potatoes each year. If you've mastered Potatoes 101, you know there are thousands of cultivated varieties of potato and 200 wild varieties. So when you want to do the mashed potato with something brand-new, besides the Idaho there are the Rose Gold, Russian Banana fingerlings, and Rose Finns, as well as red, black, and blue potatoes. And tastiest of all, perhaps, are new potatoes, which are actually younger, tender, thin-skinned versions (either white or red) of many varieties.

Super Immunity Strengths

Potatoes are in the same tuberous family as the taro root and Jerusalem artichoke, and they actually supply us with virtually all the vital nutrients we need with the exception of those two cod liver oil nutrients, vitamins A and D.

High Nutrient, Low Cal. The spuds we love have no more calories than apples (132 in a cup), and in their naked state they provide 0 grams of fat. They're loaded with both cholesterol-lowering, colon-cancer-preventing fiber and a special carbohydrate called "resistant starch," which goes through the digestive system without being absorbed at all, much like the fiber, which equals that of many whole-grain breads and cereals. In addition, potatoes contain the vitamins B_1, B_2, B_3, and B_6 for mood regulation. Potatoes are also an underappreciated source of vitamin C (providing 25 percent of your DV) and even some of that not-so-easy-to-get-from-plant-foods mineral—calcium.

Protein and Potassium. Potatoes are approximately 10 percent protein, which is twice the protein of common vegetables such as squash, peppers, and pumpkins. Potatoes also provide almost twice the feel-energized potassium of most garden-variety vegetables and fruits, such as the potassium all-stars oranges and bananas.

Taters Against Heart Attacks. In some studies, an extra 400 milligrams of potassium a day (a potato's worth) has been linked to a 40 percent reduction in the risk of heart attack. Every forkful of baked potato or spoonful of vichyssoise also delivers magnesium for energy and cardiovascular health, plus the trace minerals manganese and zinc, all of which are essential for keeping bones long and dense. Potatoes also supply modest amounts of chromium to protect against diabetes and blood sugar disorders and to suppress cravings. Last but not least, potatoes supply small amounts of the carrot phytochemicals, carotenoids, and the green tea antioxidants, polyphenols.

Healing for Whom? So who should be doubling up on the hash browns and vichyssoise for super immunity? For starters, anyone with weight or cardiovascular conditions. Both conditions are characterized by low levels of potassium and both call for calorie and fat gram counting. Potatoes, which are good examples of excellent carbohydrate foods, make high satiety value substitutes for less nutritious fattier foods. With their supply of immunity-enhancing vitamins and minerals and blood-building iron, spuds are first-rate immune boosters.

Buying, Storing, and Preparing

▶ Keep in a dark, well-ventilated place, and for long-term storage, maintain a temperature of 40°F (4°C). For short-term storage before cooking, temperatures of about 45°F to 50°F (7°C to 10°C) are best.
▶ Organic spuds trump conventionally grown spuds. Many potato crops are treated with the pesticide maleic hydrazide (also used on onions) to prevent sprouting.
▶ Taters can be stored in the crisper (high-humidity) drawer of your refrigerator. But they should be removed and kept warmer for a few days before cooking. The lower temperature turns the starch into sugar; warming allows the sugar to turn back to starch. Potatoes can keep for several months, but several weeks is the

usual shelf life. Should the potatoes start to sprout, trim before cooking.

▶ To get the most potassium out of a potato, don't boil. Researchers have found that 10 to 50 percent of the potassium in a spud may be lost when it is cooked in water. Steaming and baking reduce that loss to 3 to 6 percent.

▶ Potatoes and apples do not make good neighbors. Storing them together may alter their flavor.

▶ The cooking quality of a potato depends on its starch content. Starchy potatoes become loose and mealy when boiled or baked, but they are fine for mashing and for fries. Low-starch potatoes are dry when baked, but are good for boiling, pan-frying, and putting in scalloped dishes.

▶ Old potatoes are higher in starch and preferable to potatoes dug before they mature. Best spuds of all? The tiny culls found at roadside stands and green markets.

▶ Green skins are a red flag. A green color inside the peel indicates the presence of an excess of solanine, which in large amounts can cause headaches, nausea, diarrhea, or fatigue.

Sea Vegetables

SUPER IMMUNITY CENTERS

Sea vegetables benefit the cardiovascular, glandular, and musculo-skeletal immune centers.

There's more than fish in the sea to nourish us. Consider sea vegetables. Historically, there is evidence that sea vegetables were on the menu in Paleolithic times. Ancient Japanese and Chinese texts mention them, in Hawaii they fed the nobility nobly, and today peoples of the North Atlantic as well as of the Pacific Islands feast on everything from agar-agar to dulse and nori (the wrap around sushi) with immunity-enhancing and life-extending results.

Iodine deficiency is the most common cause of preventable brain damage. Even mild shortages can affect the thyroid gland and affect the health of the central nervous system. Are you getting your 150 micrograms RDA? You are and then some, if you're seasoning your vegetables with kelp, making your sushi with nori, and stir-frying your tofu with hijiki. A ¼-ounce serving of a sea vegetable such as dulse or hijiki may contain 4.5 milligrams, or 4,500 micrograms, of iodine, to say nothing of the vitamins, minerals, trace minerals, and antioxidants.

There are more than 160 varieties of sea vegetables (aka seaweeds) and three types—brown (kelp), red (dulse), and green (nori)—harvested from the Atlantic and Pacific Oceans for food and food additives. Although eaten more widely in Japan and China, as well as Scotland and Ireland, than here in the United States, the worldwide market is worth more than $5 billion.

Super Immunity Strengths

These large marine algae that grow in shallow waters along the ocean coastline stimulate your immune system, detoxify cells, provide calcium without saturated fat, and aid in weight loss. An unusual source of B_{12}, sea vegetables are high in carotenoids and supply all fifty-six minerals and trace minerals, such as silica and phosphorus, humans need to survive and thrive.

Weeds for Way-Down Homocysteine. A study of more than 9,000 Americans by researchers at the Center for Integrative Medicine in Tarzana, California, revealed that those with the highest intake of folate had an 86 percent lower risk for heart attack and 79 percent lower risk for stroke than those taking in less than 400 micrograms a day. Folate helps lower homocysteine, a major risk factor for stroke, and you can make your folate quota and then some by eating a little algae each day. Folate also protects you against colon and breast cancer.

Boost of B Vitamins. Under stress? Munch a little crunchy dulse to up your stress-deflecting B vitamins, especially B_{12}, which is scarce in vegetarian diets and lost as the stomach lining ages.

Detox and Revitalize DNA. Sea vegetables are a source of marine phytochemicals that help detoxify and remove heavy metals from the body. Chlorophyll (found in all the world's healthiest vegetables, especially spinach and olives) is also abundant in sea vegetables and helps reverse the damage to DNA, which is caused by cancers of the colon, breast, and lung.

Counting Calories? You'll have fewer to count if you eat hijiki instead of angel hair pasta, and use nori and dulse in place of table salt. Sea vegetables are the ideal food for dieters. The iodine and fiber they supply aid in weight loss, and as a bonus, they are alkaline forming and improve digestion.

Eat for Energy. Rich in energy-boosting minerals and trace minerals, including manganese and potassium, microalgae are fatigue erasers. Lock and load a few sea vegetables into your diet, and you may not need coffee to pick you up twice a day.

Detoxify, Strengthen Bones. Have a dulse or arame stir-fry to bolster bone density and prevent osteoporosis. Half a cup of sea vegetables offers you the calcium (in the form of calcium phosphate) in a glass of milk without the calories and the fat, plus more iron than two eggs. A bonus? It also lowers blood pressure. Hijiki is the best calcium provider among the sea vegetables. But dulse, wakame, and arame aren't far behind. To get some detoxification benefits, sprinkle everything with a little kelp, a salt and pepper substitute or flavor enhancer that has been used to treat everything from indigestion to asthma and constipation.

Anticancer. Sea vegetables are rich in calcium, iodine, and sodium alginate. They have stopped cancer growth in both test tubes and test animals, and their presence in the Japanese diet may be one reason breast cancer occurrence in Japan is well below that in the United States. Japanese scientists also believe that phytochemicals in nori fight disease-causing bacteria, prevent ulcers, and serve as an anticoagulant.

Got Hypertension? Sip a little kombu broth, or reduce your risk for stroke with kombu stew. This marine vegetable supplies healthy levels of calcium, magnesium, iron, and vitamin K.

Buying, Storing, and Preparing

▶ Buy sea vegetables in airtight packages, and transfer to airtight containers after opening.

▶ Nori, which is sold in strips and sheets, can be flash-toasted and crumbled into soups, stews, and salads.

▶ Keep a small shaker of granulated kelp, dulse, or nori on the table to use in place of salt or pepper.

▶ Cooked arame or hijiki or cooked and shredded kombu can be stirred into cooked pasta dishes or used in place of cabbage in slaws and composed salads.

▶ Add cooked diced sea vegetables to the juicer when preparing vegetable juices.

▶ Cooked leftover sea vegetables will keep two to three days in the refrigerator.

Squash

SUPER IMMUNITY CENTERS

Squash benefits the cardiovascular, digestive/detoxification, and musculoskeletal immune centers.

In Ayurvedic medicine, the squash is classified as a *sattvic* food, one that brings clarity and psychobiological well-being. Is it any wonder? There are more than forty kinds of squash (Native American for "something eaten raw"). Squash is a fruit (botanically speaking, it's a berry), but it is prepared and eaten like a vegetable and belongs to the same family as melon and cucumbers.

Super Immunity Strengths

Squashes are good sources of vitamin C (butternut is highest) and carotene. So-called winter squash (butternut, acorn, Hubbard, delicata, calabaza, spaghetti) rank after pumpkins (actually, gourdlike squash), sweet potatoes, and carrots in terms of carotene (or pro–vitamin A) content but ahead of peppers and collards. The six carotenoids (out of six hundred in nature) found most commonly in human tissue—and supplied by squash and other gourds—decrease the risk of various cancers, protect the eyes and skin from the effect of ultraviolet light, and defend against heart disease, according to the landmark Nurses' Health Study. One of them, alpha-carotene, helps slow down the aging process. Butternut is the greatest source and acorn is the lowest of this miracle nutrient for immunity.

Squashes are one of the top twelve foods for the insoluble fiber that lowers cholesterol and helps to prevent colon cancer. One cup of butternut or acorn squash provides 5 grams of total fiber, which is more than yams, brussels sprouts, or raisins. Squash seeds (especially from pumpkin) are rich in protease inhibitors that fight intestinal viruses and reproductive disorders. Dry, season, and bake them in a 400°F oven.

The name *squash* (*Curcubita pepo*) is derived from the Native American name for *gourd*, and like corn and beans, squash originated with the first Americans. (Thomas Jefferson and George Washington were squash growers and eaters.) Squash has been an essential crop in the Andes since pre-Columbian times.

Buying, Storing, and Preparing

▶ Summer squash is ready to eat when it's still immature. Buy it (or pick it) when it is small.
▶ The beta-carotene content in winter squash, which can be kept in a cool room for up to three months, increases with storage. Post-harvest squash also has a more intense flavor.
▶ Buy winter squashes that are hard, not shiny (a sign of wax or immaturity), and with a deep rich color.

Tomatoes

SUPER IMMUNITY FOODS

Tomatoes benefit the cardiovascular, nervous, glandular, and musculoskeletal immune centers.

The tomato *is* some tomato. We eat it (along with the potato) more than any other vegetable (although technically it is a fruit). Like that other favorite fruit, the apple, the tomato is complex. More than 400 compounds account for the taste of the *Solanum lycopersicum* when it is ripe, and there are 4,000 varieties of tomatoes worldwide. Shaped like grapes, potatoes, mushrooms, or grapefruit, out-of-the-mainstream heirloom tomatoes may be yellow, purple, even white or striped. We not only eat it regularly, but we also plant it in our gardens and porch planters more than any other vegetable, including squash and carrots.

Super Immunity Strengths

The French called them *pommes d'amour*, or love apples; on the other hand, they are also the symbol of the French Revolution because of their blood-red color. Today, the Mexican state of Sinaloa flies the tomato flag as its symbol. You should, too.

Cancer-Fighting Fruit. A tomato a day may keep the oncologist away. Tomatoes are rich in saponins. Also present in potatoes, soybeans, and asparagus, these plant chemicals function like natural antibiotics, warding off infection and blocking disorders such as cancer.

Big Red Risk Reducer. See red, think healthy heart. Tomatoes offer more lycopene for lowering heart disease risk than any other food source. Lycopene, the big red antioxidant that is the star of the carotenoid family and the coloring-brush compound that makes tomatoes red (or orange, purple, or black), keeps your cardio immune center well and protects against several cancers of the prostate, lung, digestive tract, cervix, and bladder like few other phytochemicals. (Out of Big Boys? You can also get your daily dose of that tomato antioxidant lycopene from watermelon and red grapefruit.) Stick with the reds for lycopene; green and yellow tomatoes are lycopene-poor.

Got Diabetes? Bump up the gazpacho and vegetable juice in your diet. Eight ounces of a tomato product daily thin the blood, according to studies reported in the *Journal of the American Medical Association*, decreasing the chance of clotting and cardiovascular problems that complicate diabetes.

Cooked Trumps Raw. While uncooked and fresh usually trumps processed, tomatoes are the exception. Curiously, cooked and canned tomato sauce and paste (yes, even ketchup) appear to offer more lycopene than a tomato out of the hand. Heating actually increases the bioavailability of lycopene, concluded a six-year study by Harvard Medical School and Harvard School of Public Health. According to reports in the *Journal of the American College of Nutrition*, the protective dose of lycopene is 35 milligrams, which is the amount in 2 cups of tomato juice or cooked tomato products. On the other hand, while cooking increases the lycopene fourfold, eating your tomato raw gives you 40 percent of what the government considers your RDA for vitamin C. Have your tomatoes both ways.

Antiaging Medicine. The tomato is some tomato when it comes to vision, too. The red-pigment antioxidant also protects against macular degeneration, the leading cause of blindness after age sixty-five, and lung damage caused by environmental toxins. When sixth-century herbalists prescribed tomatoes for cataracts, they were prescient. Lycopene and beta-carotene, as well as vitamin C, in tomatoes all help strengthen and protect vision. Tomato lycopene slows down aging by stopping free radicals from binding with oxygen, a process that slows immune building, cleansing, and repair.

Forty-Six-Plus Nutrients. Those are just the front-runner phytochemicals. Tomatoes offer forty-six more vitamins, minerals, trace minerals, and phytochemicals—chlorophyll for healthy blood, alpha-lipoic acid for improved memory and cellular integrity, tocopherols and tocotrienols (part of the vitamin E complex), as well as the flavonoids quercetin and rutin for the blood vessels and capillaries. That beefsteak, Roma, or Brandywine tomato also offers calcium, magnesium, and potassium for healthy blood pressure; the minerals zinc, iron, copper, and manganese for healthy nerves and bones; vitamin B complex for energy; and vitamin E.

To Have (a Tomato) and to Have Not. On the dark side, *Solanum lycopersicum* is also a nightshade vegetable. So if you have arthritis, tomatoes should appear infrequently at the end of your fork if at all in your diet. Nightshade vegetables also pose a problem for those whose diets are low in calcium, since tomatoes contain glycoalkaloids tomatine that can interfere with the metabolism of calcium (riper plants have less).

Buying, Storing, and Preparing

▶ To benefit the most, buy organic. According to a study in the *Journal of Agriculture and Food Chemistry*, the use of inorganic nitrogen in conventional fertilizers produces tomatoes with reduced levels of flavonoids (and what goes for tomatoes goes for potatoes and the rest of our produce). Worse, conventional tomatoes are still sprayed with fifty pesticides. One of them, the banned fungicide methyl bromide, is linked to neurological damage.

▶ Grow your own in the backyard or on the patio in pots for more flavor and nutrition than store-bought tomatoes.

▶ True vine-ripened tomatoes have twice the vitamin C and beta-carotene of tomatoes that have been ripened artificially. Be wary of where you buy tomatoes: "vine ripened" is not a legal definition. To be sure, get your store-bought tomatoes at a quality produce store.

▶ Buy them ripe. Cradled in your palm, the skin of a tomato should feel taut, as if the juices are about to burst out of the skin.

▶ To ripen tomatoes, place in a pierced paper bag with an apple or banana for several days. Don't set on a windowsill. This produces uneven ripening. The natural ethylene gases will do the rest.

▶ If it's mealy and lacks fragrance, it's been ethylene-gassed in storage. Choose vine-ripened next time or, better yet, organic—which hasn't been sprayed with any of the fifty pesticides used on tomatoes commercially.

▶ Keep your tomatoes at 60°F or higher. Temperatures below that flatten the plant's flavors and make for a pulpy texture. Store them stem-side up.

▶ Freeze those extra summer tomatoes to make them last. Blanch in hot water to remove skins, and store in freezer-safe plastic containers, leaving an inch at the top.

▶ Slice a tomato from top to bottom (not side to side) for slices that keep their juices better and longer.

▶ Heat your tomatoes (and other acidic foods) in a cast-iron skillet to maximize the amount of iron you absorb. And couple iron-rich foods with vitamin C–rich foods (i.e., beans and tomatoes, berries and cereal, spinach and lemon).

Soy Foods

SUPER IMMUNITY CENTERS

Soy foods benefit the nervous, glandular, digestive/detoxification, and musculoskeletal immune centers.

Outsourcing osteoporosis, obesity, and heart disease? Use your bean. Specifically, use your soybean. A lot of us are. Soy is the number two crop grown in the United States. Roughly 30 percent of us use soy products once a week or more, up from half that amount a decade ago. Soy (which means "wonder bean" in Chinese) has been considered a sacred grain in the Asian diet for centuries. In any one of its dozens of forms, it boosts immunity to dozens of diseases, including cancer, diabetes, obesity, heart disease, kidney disease, osteoporosis, and premature aging.

The best thing about soybeans, says the Vegetarian Resource Group, is that they count as both a vegetable and a protein. Indeed, soy is a complete protein and the only vegetable that contains more protein than carbohydrates. But that's not all that's surprising about soy. Soy foods command a shelf of their own: miso (the fermented soybean paste), tofu and tempeh (fermented soybeans), young green soybeans called edamame, soy milk, soy nuts, soy flour and soy protein powder, soy sauce, soy cheese, soy ice cream and cream, soy yogurt, soy oil and soy margarine, and soy lecithin.

Super Immunity Strengths

What can 25 grams of soy a day (the therapeutic amount) do for your immunity? Here are eight good deeds.

Build Bones and Teeth. A serving of tofu is a better source of calcium than figs, cottage cheese, or mozzarella, without the saturated fat.

Lower Cholesterol. Soybeans provide isoflavones, which are similar to the female hormone estrogen, but weaker and safer. Isoflavones are also antioxidants. The two primary isoflavones in soy, daidzein and genistein, prevent bone loss, help reduce cholesterol, and guard against various cancers. A 2006 study from the Nutrition Research Center found that eating ½ cup of cooked beans daily significantly lowers total cholesterol and LDL cholesterol.

Reduce Heart Disease. Soy contains the essential fat, linoleic acid, one of the omega-3 fatty acids, which is one reason researchers believe that eating 25 grams of soy a day can reduce your risk of becoming a victim of the number one killer, heart disease, by almost one-third.

Protect Against Breast Cancer and Prostate Cancer. The plant-based estrogens in soy prevent human estrogens from binding to receptor sites in breast tissue and causing destructive changes. Similarly, a diet rich in low-fat, high-soy foods protects against prostate cancer.

Improve Digestion. Both tofu and tempeh provide 6 grams of fiber per cup of cooked beans and are alkalizing, easy-to-digest proteins. (To be healthy, your diet should contain 80 percent alkaline foods.) This combination builds your immunity to the discomforts of constipation, hemorrhoids, and diverticulitis.

Help with Weight Loss. In a study by the Metabolic Research Group at the University of Kentucky, soy-milk meal-replacement products were more effective at triggering weight loss than dairy milk products. According to the study's author, using three meal replacements a day along with plenty of fruits and vegetables can prompt a weight loss of 30 to 50 pounds over a year.

Dial Down Diabetes. A tofu burger and a soy shake should be on the menu if you are diabetic or prediabetic. Soy is low on the glycemic index (it doesn't cause rapid hikes in insulin levels) and high in fat-free fiber (versus none for a burger), which slows down the absorption of nutrients and keeps glucose levels stable, says the National Soybean Research Laboratory.

Improve Memory, Feed the Liver. Soy lecithin—1 to 3 tablespoons a day of these sprinkle-on granules—helps cognitive function, improves liver function, and improves athletic performance, according to the Institute of Medicine of the U.S. National Academy of Sciences.

Nuts and Seeds

> Nuts and seeds benefit the glandular, digestive/detoxification, and respiratory immune centers.

Pop a nut if you know what's good for you. That handful of nuts taken five days a week may be just what you need to erase fatigue, irritability, insomnia, or asthma. At the very least, say researchers, it can reduce your risk of a heart attack by 15 percent and perhaps more. Even better, there is an inverse relationship between eating nuts and death from any cause.

Super Immunity Strengths

Nuts contain both polyunsaturated and monounsaturated fats and the essential mineral magnesium. More than 350 enzyme systems in the body depend on magnesium to function in your favor. Nuts are among the twelve food groups that are high-fiber foods—5 or more grams of fiber per serving.

Best Nuts, All-Star Seeds. While the gateway nut for many of us may be the peanut (two-thirds of our nut consumption is this legume eaten as a nut), the best choice for immunity is the walnut, followed by the almond and the pistachio. Among the seeds, sunflower and pumpkin seeds outscore sesame, chia, and all the rest, with the exception of flaxseed, in a category by itself. Pecans are rich in gamma-tocopherol, which helps minimize fat oxidation, which in turn deters arterial decline. For vitamin C, enjoy chestnuts, the only nut with any of this nutrient (3.5 ounces give you more than 40 percent of the DV for vitamin C).

Fish Oils in a Nut. Walnuts, like flaxseeds, have more antioxidants than other nuts and are one of the few sources of plant-based fatty acids (otherwise known as ALA, or alpha-linolenic acid) plus plant sterols, which help lower serum cholesterol, improve cognitive function, and reduce the risk for anxiety, depression, and Alzheimer's, says the Linus Pauling Institute. Because of this special polyunsaturated fat (or PUFA), walnuts (and walnut oil, for a treat) may also protect against asthma and rheumatoid arthritis. Walnuts are rich repositories of minerals in short supply in most diets—magnesium, folate, and copper.

Almonds for Your Health. Almonds are the best source of vitamin E among nuts, also delivering more protein (7.6 grams) than a large egg. One-quarter cup also gives you 75 percent of your need for the B vitamin biotin, essential for energy and smooth skin. Because of its argentine content, almonds promote vasodilation, relaxing the blood vessel walls and increasing blood flow.

Peanuts for Protein. One ounce of peanuts a week in some studies reduced the risk of diabetes by 30 percent. Nuts are the high point of many a hypoglycemic's day and with good reason. Like almonds, peanuts supply more protein than a large egg (without the saturated fat and cholesterol) plus fiber and zinc for normal immunity.

Pistachios for Fiber. You get more fiber from a serving of pistachios than from a half cup of spinach. You also get more nuts in a serving (47) than with most other types.

Four Heart Benefits. All nuts contain high levels of a compound called protease inhibitors, known to block cancer in animals. Also nice about nuts are the lipid-lowering polyunsaturated and monounsaturated fats they contain. In one study at Loma Linda University in California, participants who ate nuts five times a week had half the risk of heart attack and coronary-related death as those who didn't. Indeed, a handful once a week produces a 25 percent reduction in your heart disease risk, including hypertension and stroke.

Pop a Nut for Cancer Protection. Pop a big Brazil nut, and you get a small helping of selenium, a mineral that lowers the rates of several types of cancer. Stir those nuts into some steamed whole grains and you double your dose. Indeed, according to a joint report by the American Institute for Cancer Research and the World Cancer Research Fund, a high-nut diet can protect you against certain cancers—ellagic acid is one reason. Walnuts and pecans contain this phytochemical that can inactivate cancer cells and also has antiviral and antibacterial properties. Isoflavones, which protect the heart and defend the body from tumors, are another. Nuts also contain luteolin and tocotrienols.

Seeds. An ounce of sesame seeds supplies three times the iron in an ounce of beef liver without the contaminants and the fat. Hemp seeds, like quinoa and soy, supply a range of essential minerals, are a complete protein similar to milk and dairy, and are richer in omega fatty acids than olive or flaxseed oils. Seeds are available as a tasty cold-pressed oil, as a seed meal to use as a protein food, and as a ready-to-eat cereal. Keep all three on hand. See the earlier section on flaxseed, too.

Buying, Storing, and Preparing

▶ Cashews, walnuts, and other nuts can provoke allergic reactions, often severe. Also, 90 percent of kids who are allergic to tree nuts are often allergic to peanuts (a legume, not a nut) as well.

▶ Nuts are contraindicated if you have colitis, Crohn's disease, or diverticulitis.

▶ Nuts are relatively high in calories. Eat them by the handful, not like popcorn. The recommended serving is ¼ cup.

▶ Peanuts, especially when processed into peanut butter, can be contaminated with a mold that produces a highly carcinogenic substance called aflatoxin. Eat peanut butter in moderation, and buy organic to reduce the risk.

▶ Buy raw nuts in sealed packages. Roasted or exposed to light and heat (in bins), the oil in nuts can turn rancid and risky.

▶ Keep nuts and seeds in the fridge (even the freezer) to prevent rancidity. This is even truer for nut and seed oils, which should be purchased in small quantities in dark bottles to prevent oxidation from air and light.

▶ Buy cold-pressed organic nut and seed oils for safety and to get the best quality.

Whole Grains

....

> **SUPER IMMUNITY CENTERS**
>
> Whole grains benefit the digestive/detoxification, musculoskeletal, and respiratory immune centers.

The way we do anything is the way we do everything, yoga masters tell us. Just so. Take bread, for example: are you the "spelt today, sprouted rye tomorrow" type? Or the "white bread all the time" type? Only 5 percent of the grain foods in our diet are whole grains. If you're typical, you're eating only half the whole grains you really need to keep all your immune centers firing. Plenty of us have a half-baked diet. Fewer than 8 percent of adults get three or more whole-grain servings daily. But swap that white rice for brown basmati or quinoa, for example, and make that wrap whole wheat, and you could start lowering your stroke risk by as much as 50 percent, suggests studies such as the Nurses' Health Study.

Whole grains mean a lot more than wheat these days, no matter how you slice it. To get your whole grains, enjoy wheat, rye, barley, oats, amaranth, buckwheat, corn, and quinoa.

Super Immunity Strengths

Eating the whole grain (bran, germ, and endosperm) version of whatever it is under your peanut butter, curry, or steamed vegetables helps prevent several cancers, diabetes, high cholesterol, and weight gain, in addition to strokes. Grains can give you a longer lease on life. According to the Iowa Women's Health Study, women who ate at least one serving of a whole grain daily lowered their overall mortality risk by 14 to 19 percent. In a similar study of Finnish men, eating more whole-grain rice tracked with fewer deaths from all causes.

Some whole grains do it—lengthen your life, protect your heart, prevent cancer—a whole lot better than others. Rice, barley, couscous, and oats are all low-GI (glycemic index) foods, which means they have minimal effects on blood sugar and insulin (unlike high-GI offenders like baked potatoes and white bread).

The Whole Truth
- Most grains are actually grasses. One family includes wheat, rye, barley, and oats; a second group includes amaranth and buckwheat.
- Corn is actually a grass that we eat as a vegetable.
- Quinoa is an herb eaten like a grain.
- Only two grains—amaranth and quinoa—are complete proteins, providing all sixteen amino acids just like dairy and meat.
- Oats contain more fat (polyunsaturated and monounsaturated) than any other grain.

EMS for LDL. Hypertension, the most important risk factor for a stroke, happens less often to those who keep their fiber up. In grains, that fiber comes bound up with vitamin E, a major nutrient for preventing stroke and lowering homocysteine, another coronary risk factor. Highest scores for fiber go to triticale (8.7 g per ¼ cup serving), barley (8 g), and amaranth (7.4 g). Brown rice scores 0.9 (but that's still five times the fiber of white rice). The fiber in barley contains beta-glucans, which are polysaccharides (also found in mushrooms, oats, and yeast) that activate immune cells, lower cholesterol, slow aging, and fight cancer.

Oats, Barley, and Diabetes. Polishing off three servings of whole grains daily protects you against developing type 2 diabetes by improving insulin sensitivity. In tests, fasting insulin was in fact 10 percent lower when unrefined grains like oats, barley, and wheat were on the menu. Make it barley, and you get chromium, important for keeping blood glucose stable.

Good Gut Reactions. Grains high in insoluble fiber, like spelt and rye, help prevent conditions like IBS and gallstones. Rye, brown rice, and other grains are also rich in lignans, which establish a healthy flora in the intestines, and these in turn are prescriptive for breast and other cancers and heart disease.

Fewer Pounds, More Protein. Have some quinoa (pronounced "keen-wa") with that reduced-calorie fruit salad. This millet-sized seed is a complete protein, containing all sixteen amino acids, and it has more satiety value (i.e., fills you up) than the rice or wheat you usually eat.

Buying, Storing, and Preparing

▶ Most grains can be prepared like rice. Rinse first, cover with water, bring to a boil, reduce to a simmer, and cook until soft. Use a two-to-one ratio for quinoa, amaranth, millet, and buckwheat; use a three-to-one ratio for oats and barley. Use too much water rather than too little. You can always pour off any excess.

▶ Get organic when you can. The toxic chemical sulfuryl fluoride is used as a pesticide when storing conventional grains, fruit, and nuts.

▶ Avoiding gluten? That still leaves flours, breads, and crackers made from millet, amaranth, quinoa, corn, teff, and flours made from beans like soybeans and chickpeas.

▶ To shorten the cooking time of whole grains, toast first or presoak.

Yogurt

....

> Yogurt benefits the nervous, digestive/detoxification, and muscu-
> loskeletal immune centers.

Did you know that if you're the average American eater you will consume a total of twenty tons of food during your lifetime? This job is
made possible only because of the trillions of bacteria in your gut.
Actually, there are more probiotics than cells in the human body.
There are a total of 2.2 pounds of probiotics in your gastrointestinal
tract. These tiny organisms, the chief reason most of us eat yogurt,
support healthy digestion and immune function, ease allergies, tame
inflammation, lower cholesterol, eliminate bad bacteria such as *E. coli*,
and lots more. Who could ask for anything more?

Super Immunity Strengths

Consider calcium. You get 35 to 40 percent of your daily value (DV)
from a cup of cultured milk (i.e., yogurt). There are 389 milligrams of
calcium per cup, more than in a cup of low-fat or skim milk. Even better for skeletal health, that cultured milk comes packaged with bone-
building vitamin K and phosphorus.

More Calcium, Less Lactose. Consider the lactose factor. Some 50
million of us are lactose-intolerant. But yogurt, because of its reduced
lactose (milk sugar), is often tolerated. (The bacteria consume much
of the milk sugar.) If even this doesn't make dairy more gut-palatable,
there is always sheep yogurt, goat yogurt, soy yogurt, even rice and
oat yogurt out there. What's the dose that does it? For maintenance,
pick a product that delivers 1 to 2 billion colony-forming units (cfu)
daily. To recolonize the intestines after a bout of antibiotics, for example, you need 10 billion cfu each day for fourteen days.

Is it any wonder the French call yogurt "the milk of eternal life"? It should certainly add a year or two to yours if you take it seriously and spoon it up regularly.

Seven Reasons Yogurt Should Be One of Your One-a-Day Foods

1. Yogurt bacteria help tame inflammation in arthritis, suppress the bacteria *H. pylori* that triggers ulcers, and reduce the odor-causing bacteria in halitosis.
2. In human studies, yogurt daily for a month improved the ratio of LDL to HDL cholesterol, as well as lowered homocysteine levels. Also, in some animal studies it helped decrease tumor activity in colon cancer.
3. A regular intake of this microorganism-rich food can help clear up your complexion. (Use it as a moisturizer externally.)
4. Yogurt is good preventive medicine for vaginal yeast infections, thrush, and vaginitis in women.
5. *L. acidophilus* (one of the good bacteria found in all true yogurts) provides a hostile environment for disease-causing bacteria such as *Salmonella*, *Listeria*, and other types of toxins that cause food poisoning. Yogurt triggers your immune center to make more antibodies and slows the growth of harmful bacteria by as much as 75 percent.
6. Yogurt protects you from diarrhea, dysentery, and cholera, as well as everyday gas and bloating.
7. Yogurt may be a tool in the fight against colon cancer, according to the National Cancer Institute. Harvard Medical School researchers say yogurt is especially effective against women's reproductive cancers.

Yogurtlike products also deserve space in your fridge. Other probiotic foods include kefir (read labels for sugar content before buying flavored varieties), miso, sauerkraut, and some cheeses.

Buying, Storing, and Preparing

▶ Look for brands with the "live and active cultures" seal from the National Yogurt Association. These products must contain 100 million live bacteria per gram at the time of manufacture. Look for the expiration date no more than 10 days ahead.

▶ Buy organic to avoid the genetically modified animal growth hormone rBGH used in much commercial dairy milk (it's not required to be listed among the ingredients).

▶ Try the new specialty yogurts such as Activia and DanActive, which guarantee they contain the number of organisms listed on the label (the well-researched *B. animalis* and *L. casei*).

▶ Eat your yogurt with some prebiotic fiber for maximum benefits. Prebiotics are soluble dietary fibers that stimulate the growth of good bacteria. Look for FOS, XOS, GOS, or inulin among the ingredients.

▶ Try a super-yogurt like kefir (a type of fermented milk), which can offer 3 billion bacteria per serving.

▶ Aged cheeses like cheddar and blue are also rich in good bacteria—usually 3 to 10 million, depending on the length of aging.

IMMUNITY BUSTERS

~

Eating for Thirteen Health Conditions That Compromise Immunity

C ERTAIN FOODS CAN HELP supersize your immunity and protect you from both acute and chronic complaints such as allergies, arthritis, fatigue, and even heart disease and diabetes. If you're already down and out, those same foods can improve and speed up recovery.

Acne and Other Skin Disorders

Acne affects the glandular and digestive/detoxification immune centers.

Give peas a chance if you have acne, psoriasis, eczema, rosacea, or any other dermatological disorders or just want to avoid them all. Green peas, black beans, red tomatoes, and all vibrantly colored foods top the list of skin-healing foods. Color is the key to nutrient density and Oxygen Radical Absorbance Capacity (ORAC) value; foods with high ORAC values are high in antioxidants.

Acne, an inflammatory skin disorder characterized by pimples, whiteheads, and blackheads afflicts not just teens but as much as 80 percent of the population at one time or another. Acne is the result of not simply poor skin hygiene, but more often of overactive oil glands. Inflammation—indicating a blip in the workings of one or more of the body's immune centers—can be triggered by a genetic predisposition, PMS, the use of oral contraceptives, *Candidiasis*, food allergies, certain medications (including thyroid medications, steroids, and immunosuppressive drugs), hormonal imbalances, and nutritional deficiencies, as well as by a diet high in saturated and hydrogenated fats or an imbalanced pH (too acid or too alkaline)—not to mention excess dietary iodine, which irritates pores. (Iodine source foods include iodized salt, shellfish, and fast foods, the biggest offender.) One of the problems, according to the American Academy of Dermatology, is that the skin (your body's biggest organ) functions as an emergency detoxification organ, and when the liver and kidneys are overtaxed, the skin takes over. But this handoff can cause dermatological conditions such as acne, psoriasis, and beyond. Here's what to do about it.

What to Eat

If hormone imbalance is the problem, or part of it, more zinc and omega-3-rich foods and supplements can help reboot your metabolism.

It's also possible that you're a victim of dermatological insulin resistance, meaning you don't process sugar well. This causes surface bacteria to convert sugar to acne-causing acid. Accentuate the positive: go on a sugar fast to test out the possibility; then eliminate the negative (all sugars).

Get some shut-eye. Acne and other conditions are often the result of poor sleep and poor hygiene, as well as stress. Nighttime savasana rejuvenates the skin, allowing the lymphatic system to drain off toxins and recharge the immune system.

Skin disruptions can be calmed by increasing soups (and other juicy foods) that plug vitamin A (and beta-carotene), vitamin B complex, fiber, zinc, and enzymes into your diet, plus vitamin C foods that fight free-radical skin damage caused by the sun, pollution, cigarettes, and more. (Did you know that your chin may also break out if your digestive system is out of balance? The jawline and chin correspond to the intestinal region, say traditional Chinese medicine practitioners.)

Beans, peas, tomatoes, watermelon, pink grapefruit, and other foods that supply the carotenoid lycopene help stabilize cell membranes and restore the skin's integrity under the sun. Eat plenty of melon, squash, carrots, spinach, parsley, cucumbers, and cabbage-family vegetables. The ascorbic and caffeic acids in cukes soothe and reduce inflammation. (Cukes also supply fiber for your heart and potassium and magnesium to lower blood pressure.)

Add herbs with high antioxidant value such as oregano and marjoram. Don't forget leafy greens for folate, which protects you from trace amounts of arsenic. In very small amounts, arsenic can cause skin disorders as well as cancer, diabetes, and coronary disease.

Water is also EMS for the epidermal wellness (which is one reason soup is such a skin saver). Drink six to eight glasses of filtered water daily, and use some of it to wash down a daily supplement of acidophilus- and bifidus-friendly bacteria (especially if you're on acne-fighting antibiotics or steroid meds that destroy friendly bacteria). For more probiotic power, include yogurt or yogurt whips, dips, drinks, or yogurt-based soups three times a week.

When used externally, all teas suppress inflammation that leads to outbreaks, and when taken internally, especially stinging nettle or cleavers tea, they fight free radicals. The calcium and folic acid they supply reduce swelling and redness.

What Not to Eat: Foods to Subtract

What you *don't* put on your plate or in your bowl matters, too. Decrease your intake of processed foods, refined foods, red meat (a source of inflammatory arachidonic acid), refined carbohydrates (especially refined sugar), starchy foods, salt, and alcohol to improve your face value.

Consider Sensitivities. Food allergies can be a contributing cause of dermatitis, and sensitivity to gluten (celiac disease) is common in victims of skin disorders. Check it out by eliminating sources of gluten (wheat, rye, barley, oats, spelt, bran, wheat germ) from your diet like bread and pasta for a week. Or have your heath care provider administer a diagnostic test for celiac disease. Dairy products are also frequent offenders. Even if you aren't lactose intolerant, Harvard University researchers warn about a link between dairy products and acne, possibly because of the hormones and bioactive ingredients in cow's milk, cheese, and ice cream.

Arthritis

....

Arthritis affects the nervous and musculoskeletal immune centers.

Rheumatism and rain do not go together, despite the old wives' tale. But super immunity foods and sore joints do. And you're right as rain if you reach for a spoonful of Mustard Greens Pesto (see page 142) or Olive-Oil Mayonnaise (see page 143) when your joints are jumping, either from rheumatoid arthritis (RA) or osteoarthritis (OA).

Contrary to conventional folk wisdom, arthritis ("fire in the joints") is really little affected by the thermometer. So if you are one of the millions of Americans with one of the more than one hundred forms of what is known by the umbrella term *arthritis*, you can leave the umbrella home when you are symptomatic and think guacamole, grilled tofu, toasted walnuts, and garlic sauce.

Arthritis is the result of inflammatory compounds known as prostaglandins (a kind of hormone) disturbing cell membranes' health and integrity, producing pain and impaired movement. Arthritis can strike any joint, causing stiffness, pain, and deterioration as cartilage breaks down. Most commonly affected areas are joints of the thumb, fingers, neck, toes, hips, knees, and lower back. Sad to say, what is often the first line of defense—aspirin, ibuprofen, and steroids— should be the last, since these medications only mask the discomfort; deplete other nutrients important for proper immune function, such as folic acid, iron, potassium, vitamin C, zinc, and vitamin B complex; and even promote further damage. (If you take them, take the nutritional supplement resveratrol, too, to reduce risk.)

But anti-inflammatory foods plus targeted supplements, specific exercises, and other smart strategies can make all the difference between easy living and compromised movement. Preventing and healing arthritis is a matter of what you do and don't eat, as well as what you do and don't do.

What to Eat

There are plenty of low-allergen options for the joint-healing bowl and plate, especially whole-grain breads and pastas (look for the new multigrain pastas using bean and oat flours), carrots, cabbage, lettuce, olives, and olive oil. Avocados and soybeans both supply unsaponifiable oil (ASU). Joints also need a good supply of potassium-rich foods, so think spinach, broccoli, sea vegetables, and soybean miso. Broccoli and zucchini also supply salicylates, which turn off COX-2 enzymes, which in turn triggers inflammation. Onions and garlic supply joint-feeding sulphur (found in joints supporting muscles, tendons, and ligaments) or methylsulfonylmethane (MSM), also found in some fruits, vegetables, grains, sunflower seeds, lentils, garlic, and yogurt. To absorb MSM better, take with vitamin C and vitamin C–rich foods.

Anti-Inflammatory Foods. Walnuts provide inflammation-taming omega-3 fatty acids; pineapple supplies the anti-inflammatory and anti-allergen enzyme bromelain. Other raw, steamed, or juiced foods that boost joint well-being include cherries and dark berries, grapes, brussels sprouts, and mustard greens. The curcumin found in turmeric used in curry powder (and also sold as a supplement) is another natural anti-inflammatory.

The microalgae spirulina supplies phycocyanins that help decrease arthritic flare-ups and protect cartilage (as well as the essential fatty acid gamma-linolenic acid [GLA]). Try a scoop of spirulina powder stirred into vegetable juice or yogurt every day.

More Water, More Tea. Drink up. Joint cartilage, which acts as a cushion between joints and surrounding bones, is 75 to 80 percent water. Soup is an important lubricant, along with water, followed by herbal teas and fresh juices. Rosehip tea provides vitamin C and bioflavonoids; in high doses as a supplement, it relieves pain and improves range of motion.

Get Plenty of Vitamin D. Osteoarthritis is linked to low vitamin D levels. A chronic shortfall of this nutrient can lead to chronic muscle and joint pain, even hypertension and osteoporosis. Eighty percent of all back pain victims are vitamin-D-deficient, say experts. In a study of more than 30,000 middle-aged women over an eleven-year span, those taking vitamin D supplements were 34 percent less prone to RA. Soak up the sun and include plenty of vitamin D source foods in your diet—egg yolks and oily fish or cod liver oil (if you eat them), and even mushrooms that have been exposed to ultraviolet (UV) light are sources of vitamin D, along with ten to fifteen minutes of unfiltered sunlight daily. (SPF 8 sunblock reduces vitamin D production in the body by 95 percent.) Sunlight also increases production of serotonin, which helps turn off pain.

What Not to Eat: Foods to Subtract

Avoid Saturated Fats. Don't use saturated fats found in animal products that cause an accumulation of inflammation-accelerating arachidonic acid in the tissues. In addition, people with arthritis are often allergic to both meat and dairy. Trans fats still found in many processed foods are another *don't*.

Avoid the Nightshades. The Foundation for Integrated Medicine in New York City estimates that 25 percent of OA sufferers have food allergies—some of those sensitivities may be to the nightshade family vegetables, including eggplant, tomatoes, peppers, and potatoes. (Tobacco, besides what it does to the rest of the body, is also a nightshade member and threatens joints as well.) Other problem foods that may exacerbate symptoms include fatty fish, egg yolks, coffee, and dairy products and sugar.

Allergies

> Allergies affect the nervous, glandular, digestive/detoxification, and respiratory immune centers.

If you're sneezing and wheezing, put down the tissues and pick up your soup spoon or salad fork. A Caesar salad or cream of mushroom soup is nothing to sneeze at if you're trying to kick-start your immune response, manage your pollen and food-elevated histamine levels, or soothe irritated membranes, nerves, or mood. Other soup and salad ingredients on the immunity A-list: decongesting ginger, peppers, onions, and fresh herbs and spices.

Food allergy, which may be the leading cause of all undiagnosed symptoms, was first noted by Hippocrates, who linked milk with gastric upset. Of course, it's possible to be allergic to almost anything we breathe, eat, drink, or touch (sight and hearing are exempt senses). Allergies to pollen, pork, peanuts, or perfume can affect any part of the body, producing mildly irritating symptoms such as sneezing or more severe autoimmune disorders such as arthritis or celiac disease. Thirty-seven million Americans also have sinusitis, and untreated, it can lead to asthma. (Some naturopathic doctors believe that all inhalation allergies actually arise from food allergies.)

The culprits are countless—your genetic inheritance (there's a 67 percent chance you'll be allergic if both of your parents were) and, some believe, environmental toxins, for example. Others theorize that allergies are the result of accumulated toxins, including heavy metals, in the body.

Overconsumption of a limited number of foods and ingredients (especially the top six offender foods: corn, soy, milk, citrus, eggs, and wheat) are also problematic. If you have a wheat sensitivity, an allergy to wheat, or full-blown celiac disease (gluten intolerance), you may experience anything from headaches and sinus congestion to bloating, itching, and depression with every slice of toast or soup-borne crouton.

Allergens enter the body through the mucous membranes of the nose and are absorbed by the intestinal tract through the skin. The integrity of your immune system is key. A malfunctioning immune system and unchecked stress can trigger allergies. Allergies (including asthma) can even develop as a side effect of *Candidiasis* (yeast infection), which can itself develop in response to a lengthy regimen of steroids or antibiotics.

Antibiotics can also increase your body's sensitivity to common allergens, so use them conservatively and only when absolutely necessary. Various combinations of the above factors—stress plus asthma, for example, or yeast infection and food allergy, or asthma plus an antibiotics regimen—make any allergic profile all the more confounding.

What to Eat

Don't short yourself on the essentials. Allergies can appear early or late in life as a result of nutritional deficiencies, especially a shortage of essential fatty acids (such as the omega-3s found in flax, hemp, and sea vegetables), which weakens the immune system. What you see or feel isn't necessarily what you've got. An allergy to apples, for example, may really be a reaction to the pesticide residues on the apple or to the processing involved in turning apples into applesauce, rather than a reaction to the apple itself. Test it out when in doubt. Or better yet, stick to organic produce to protect yourself.

Nutritional self-defense can begin with any omega-3-rich food. In German studies, people who consumed the most omega-3-rich foods had the lowest rates of hay fever. Keep nonanimal source foods such as flaxseed, walnuts, hempseed oil, soy foods, and sea greens in the kitchen, and have two or more daily. If you eat fish, wild salmon is another good source.

Soups, salads, juices supplying fresh fruits (including citrus, if tolerated), fresh vegetables (especially carrots, celery, beets, and cucumber), as well as seeds and nuts and low-fat proteins stimulate antibody production. Carrots, celery, dill, parsley, and fennel, all members of the carrot family, are low- to no-allergen foods. Note that ragweed sufferers may be sensitive to bananas, cucumbers, melons, zucchini, sunflower seeds, and chamomile tea (cooking sometimes reduces the effect of the offending allergen). Garlic, ginger, cayenne, and onions stimulate production of IGA, an antibody in the gastrointestinal tract that can prevent absorption of allergens.

Natural Antihistamines. Vitamin C is a natural antihistamine. Vitamin C source foods are EMS for both environmental as well as food allergies. This means eating citrus, broccoli, kiwi, cabbage, sea vegetables, and also foods rich in beta-carotene and vitamin A to strengthen mucous membranes. Drink ginger broth or ginger tea (it also settles the stomach) and up your intake of pungent foods to clear nasal passages. Foods that contain the bioflavonoid quercetin—apples, onions (sweet ones like Vidalia onions can be eaten raw like apples), and bananas—can diminish the inflammation that causes sinus pain and congestion. Nutritional yeast, mushrooms, oats, and barley all contain small amounts of beta-glucan, a polysaccharide that can activate a powerful immune response. For a higher dose, add a beta-glucan supplement.

Bioflavonoids found in rosehip and green teas, red wine, and most fruits prevent the release of histamine, while zinc (found in whole grains, pumpkin seeds, and legumes) boosts immunity. Adding herbs, which produce fewer or no allergic reactions, can boost that healing power. Rosemary helps with sinusitis and asthma, especially coupled with other culinary herbs like basil or marjoram.

The Common Cold

> The common cold affects the glandular, digestive/detoxification, and respiratory immune centers.

"I like good soup, not fine words," said Molière, good advice that goes double if you have a cold, which ranks as humanity's leading physical illness. Besides rest, stress reduction, high-level hygiene, and plenty of fluids, eating nutrient-dense salads, fruits, and vegetables can be part of the protocol that pulls you through. You'll need all three, in fact, if you spend the typical ten to fourteen days with a rhinoviral infection.

The common cold (so called because year in, year out there are one billion cases of it) can make you uncommonly uncomfortable. Symptoms include (but are not limited to) head and nasal congestion, sore throat, coughing, sneezing, watery eyes, aches and pains, and fatigue, and a slight fever is also a possibility. The window of opportunity for getting or escaping a cold is also slight. The virus gains entry to your body usually by attaching itself to the back of the adenoid area. It manifests itself eighteen to twenty-four hours later, keeping you contagious for five days after. The rhinovirus can remain live for eighteen hours on hard surfaces. The cold is a close cousin of more serious and potentially chronic conditions, including bronchitis, sinusitis, otitis media, and influenza. The flu is a winter phenomenon because of cold air and relative humidity. Dry air enables the virus to be airborne longer. The respiratory system also works more slowly, say researchers, during the dry winter season. It's nothing to sniff at and reason enough to become immune-food savvy.

What to Eat

Anti-Inflammatory Vegetables. Your get-better bowl or plate doesn't have to be filled with chicken soup either. According to recent studies, the miraculous "chicken soup effect" is not due to chicken at all, but to the anti-inflammatory action of the vegetables that go with it, such as onions, garlic, carrots, parsnips, and everyday parsley. As a bonus, these are all alkalizing foods that help the body defend against pathogens. Ideally, the body should be 75 percent alkaline and 25 per cent acid. (Acid foods that can make a bad situation like a cold worse include cheese, coffee, sugar, and animal proteins.)

In fact, from see-through broths to chunky chowders, soup is a superior delivery service for the breathe-easy nutrients that restore the integrity of the respiratory system (lungs, sinuses, throat). All soups help thin the mucus in the bronchial tube, but some are especially formulated to ease or even reverse a cold by supplying the key nutrients that help mobilize the killer white blood cells that a virus depresses or incapacitates. In each bowl, you get vitamin C (plus bioflavonoids), which can reduce cold symptoms up to 30 percent; vitamin A, in the form of beta-carotene, to strengthen and safeguard the mucous membrane; zinc, which directly attacks the rhinoviruses in the tissues of the throat and the mouth; amino acids, which provide protein for healing; and allium, the sulphurous detoxifying compound found in garlic and onions. What's the dosage for these soups when you're sick? It's up to you. Depending on the stability of your stomach, try downing three or more mugs or glasses, diluting the serving with filtered water when needed. If need be, ingest less and inhale more—you'll still benefit.

Berry Up. Berries are the number one source of antioxidants in the diet. Eat all kinds, spoon them on cereals, or juice them.

Depression

. . . .

> Depression affects the nervous, glandular, and digestive/detoxification immune centers.

If you're down in your cups, maybe you need a bowl of mood-elevating minestrone or a Bitter Greens Salad (see page 152). And don't hold back on those complex-carbohydrate vegetables like carrots, potatoes, and tomatoes. According to researchers at the Massachusetts Institute of Technology (MIT), carbohydrates are the key to stimulating serotonin, the neurotransmitter that helps boost mood and feelings of satiety. The brain makes serotonin only after it has been fed carbs with little or no protein. (Interestingly, women naturally have less serotonin than men and twice the incidence of depression.) The other four transmitters that must be firing for you to feel good are dopamine, melatonin, epinephrine, and norepinephrine—all supplied by foods such as whole grains, beans, and greens, which should be embedded in our meal plans.

We need all the great soups, salads, slaws, and stir-fries we can get. According to the World Health Organization (WHO), by 2020 depression will surpass cancer as the second leading cause of death and disability in the United States. Currently, fifteen million of us are blue—and that's bad. Long-term depression can alter DNA patterns and increase your risk of cancer and heart disease.

Of course, maybe it's not a few neurotransmitters but the whole family tree that's failing you. If your first-degree parent was depressed, there's a 25 to 30 percent chance that you will be, too. Impaired blood flow to the brain can put you at risk for depression, and so can anemia and low thyroid function. (Women are 50 percent more likely than men to develop hypothyroidism, which often manifests as depression.)

Depression can be the upshot of a shortage of adrenal and DHEA hormones as well as the sex hormones testosterone, estrogen, and progesterone. But before you pop a pill, have your health care provider

IMMUNITY BUSTERS: Eating for Thirteen Health Conditions   83 •

run a hormone panel (blood test). Are you hypoglycemic? Chronic low blood sugar levels can trigger the blues. Go from three squares a day to six small, well-balanced minimeals to keep the brain nourished in a time-released fashion.

Allergies Are Triggers

Eliminating foods that you are allergic or sensitive to can improve mood. Wheat and dairy products are especially problematic. Eliminating sugar and artificial sweeteners can help (switch to healthier substitutes such as stevia and Xylitol). If you're bending an elbow, do it with dumbbells, not cocktails. Alcohol depletes the brain of mood-stabilizing omega-3 fatty acids (as well as interferes with the absorption of nutrients in general). Remember, the brain has a higher metabolic rate than the muscles and a greater need for nutrients. One nutrient that is poorly absorbed and in short supply in the American diet is magnesium. Upping your intake can take you from sulky to smiley. Snack on almonds, enjoy spinach pie, have oatmeal for breakfast, and eat potatoes for lunch; nonvegetarians can add halibut, a good source of magnesium. High levels of homocysteine in the blood can produce depressive symptoms, too. Bring the levels down with doses of vitamin B_6, B_{12}, and folic acid. Oral contraceptives, which deplete vitamin B_6 and the amino tyrosine needed for cerebral stability, also can produce depressive symptoms.

The SAD-Sad Connection

What if you're sad because of SAD? There are plenty of natural ways to beat seasonal affective disorder (SAD). Try the homeopathic remedies sepia, aurum metallicum, or phosphorus. Or consider Ayurvedic self-massage called *Sarvabhyanga,* which uses vigorous upward strokes from the feet to the head to rebalance energy and mood. Also, try getting up early and taking a walk in the early morning light for 30 minutes, or get yourself a light box to make up for the missing sunlight, essential for vitamin D production.

Don't forget, the higher your body burden of chemicals, the likelier you'll feel melancholy, sad, or depressed. The hormones in meat; the PCBs in fish; the arsenic, fluoride, and stray pharmaceuticals in water; air pollution; exposure to pesticides; and volatile chemicals in cosmetics, clothes, and furniture all impact the *brain*.

What to Eat: Blues Busters

So what's in the blues-busting bowl, plate, or cup? Think of foods, hot or cold, thick or thin, with ingredients that will keep your digestive tract healthy, since that's where 99 percent of your neurotransmitters are located (only 1 percent are in the brain). Foods that will safely boost serotonin include whole-grain breads and pastas, yams, potatoes, squashes, and root vegetables, including ginger, carrots, turnips, radishes, and celery root. Remember, vibrantly colored foods are rich in antioxidants, which protect the brain from oxidative damage. The two nonanimal foods that may do the most for brain health, according to researchers, are spinach and blueberries.

These good carbohydrate foods elevate the amino acid tryptophan, which in turn raises serotonin. The right soup, stew, or shake also helps elevate the amino acid dopamine, which when balanced, produces good moods, mental clarity, and high energy. Nonanimal amino-acid foods include tofu, dried beans, nuts, and nutritional yeast. Remember, for best results, the proteins you eat should be low in fat to reduce toxin intake and lower calories.

Better Foods, Better Moods. More bean burgers can mean a better mood because even a mild deficiency of iron (a star ingredient in dried beans) can affect mood, memory, and energy. Make or look for foods rich in iron and vitamin C, and the soups that contain them, including dried beans, lentils, citrus, and leafy dark greens. Greens—the darker the better—in your soup and salad bowl can help block mental decline when it manifests as depression, say researchers at the James A. Haley VA Medical Center in Tampa. The antioxidants in greens block free radicals that can cause brain fog.

Lots of fresh and organic fruits and vegetables also keep brain cells nourished and functioning, along with the energizing vitamin-B-complex foods, such as dairy (if you eat it, make it organic) and soy foods. High-quality amino acids from nuts, seeds, legumes, and soy foods, along with vitamin B complex (especially B_6 and B_{12}), create a starting block for the production of neurotransmitters. Peas, beans, nuts and seeds, and avocado also supply brain-energizing vitamin B_1 and inositol. Taking extra B vitamins and essential fatty acids (EFAs) can encourage the brain to regenerate itself. Herbs and spices to improve mood and brain function include ginger, fennel, dill, basil, and coriander.

Fat for the Brain. The brain is 50 percent fat, and you need to feed it a minimum of 2 grams of EFAs a day to feel up. Get EFAs through foods such as flax, hemp, walnuts, and sea greens, or take omega-3 supplements to prevent depression, mood swings, and memory slides. Peanuts, grapes, and berries supply resveratrol, a powerful protector of brain tissue. Add a supplement to get a therapeutic dose. Resveratrol is also found in red wine—choose organic to avoid processing toxins such as sulfites.

What Not to Eat: Foods to Subtract

Switch from regular coffee (caffeine stimulates the central nervous system) to green tea, which supplies brain-protective polyphenols called catechins. Add lemon juice to couple with vitamin C for more insurance.

Diabetes

Diabetes affects the cardiovascular, glandular, musculoskeletal, and respiratory immune centers.

Chicken soup may be good for the common cold, but onion soup is just what the dietician ordered for diabetes. Both onions and garlic are rich in blood-sugar-lowering compounds and provide vitamins C and E, two nutrients that diabetics are commonly low in. Eating therapeutically is a habit that takes practice, and it pays if you're diabetic. All you need is your soup spoon, salad fork, tea cup, and some face time with fresh foods, including raw fruits and vegetables, that improve your chances of resisting or rebounding from this disorder.

Diabetes, a condition of elevated blood sugar, affects 40 percent of the population, and it's climbing by 6 percent yearly. According to the American Dietetic Association, by 2010, diabetes will become the leading cause of death in the United States. Diabetes is characterized by a disturbance of the pancreatic hormone insulin. When insulin builds up in the blood instead of being taken up into the cells, a state of hyperglycemia (high blood sugar) results. This can lead to damaged blood vessels and then to heart, eye, or kidney disease. There are two major forms of this disease: diabetes type 1 (juvenile onset) and diabetes type 2 (adult onset). The latter is the more common of the two, affecting 90 to 95 percent of the afflicted, many of whom are unaware that they are affected. Insulin is always required for type 1, but not always for type 2.

People with diabetes are more prone to cardiovascular disease because of faulty fat metabolism; may have poor circulation due to the narrowing of blood vessels, which leads to many complications; and have a heightened susceptibility to infection. In addition, 90 percent of those with diabetes are overweight or obese. A poor diet high in fiber-depleted simple carbohydrates, unmanaged food allergies, and frequent viral infections can all make matters worse. Stress can cause adrenaline levels to rise, triggering a hike in blood sugar. Life expectancy is typically four to eight years shorter for diabetics compared to nondiabetics.

What to Eat

Your diabetes immunity-boosting defense kit should include frequent helpings of soups, salads, and other dishes formulated from low-fat, high-fiber beans, fresh fruits, and fresh vegetables, whose pectin content reduces the need for insulin and lowers blood sugar. According to the U.S. Food and Drug Administration (FDA), Americans, especially diabetics, should eat more than the ½ cup of beans they currently consume a week and shoot for a much-higher-in-fiber goal of 3 cups a week. Beans are low in total fat, with no saturated fat, but have important nutrients such as calcium, iron, folic acid, and potassium. Beans help lower the risk of hypertension and stroke as well as helping manage diabetes, says the FDA. In fact, a low-fat plant-based diet actually helps repair the way the body uses insulin rather than just compensating for the malfunctioning of this hormone, says the Physicians Committee for Responsible Medicine (PCRM).

Whole Grains for Healing. Add three or more helpings of whole grains daily, and you reduce your chances of worsening insulin resistance or of developing Metabolic Syndrome, that cluster of factors that often precedes type 2 diabetes. Whole grains are a source of chromium, and this trace mineral is required for insulin to act on cells, moving glucose from the blood into the cells. Insulin resistance, which is at the root of type 2 diabetes, might in fact be related to chromium deficiency, which is widespread, say researchers at Wake Forest University School of Medicine in Winston-Salem, North Carolina. In test animals, increased chromium increased life span, lowered blood pressure, and normalized hemoglobin levels. Eating refined foods, which are low in chromium, also increases chromium loss from the body.

Watch the GI. Keep an eye on the glycemic index (GI), which can tell you how rapidly a carbohydrate turns into glucose. In the Nurses' Health Study, a one-third drop in risk came from eating a low-GI-foods diet with plenty of cereal fiber. (See glycemicindex.com for details.) Try some unusual low-sugar, low-glycemic-index fruits such as papaya, Asian pear, quince, star fruit, and the pomelo, a giant citrus.

Normalizing Blood Sugar with Your Knife and Fork. That kit for normalizing blood sugar should also include berries (with blueberries at the top of the shopping list), sweet potatoes (which help control

C-reactive protein in the blood, as a bonus), vitamin-B-complex-rich nutritional yeast, soybeans, sea vegetables, and dairy or nondairy yogurt, plus eggs, if you eat them. Plus, include antioxidant-rich all-star eats such as oranges and other citrus, tomatoes, squash, spinach, and both onions and garlic (the more, the better, since both contain blood-sugar-lowering sculpture compounds). Potatoes, yeast, and spinach contain small amounts of alpha-lipoic acid, an antioxidant that improves insulin sensitivity and blood sugar control (as well as repairs cartilage). So do mono- and polyunsaturated oils such as flaxseed, rapeseed, and olive oils.

Look for bitter melon (aka balsam pear) in the ethnic foods section or fresh produce section of your market or in Asian food marts. Steamed or sautéed with beans or another ingredient to offset its bitterness, it contains a polypeptide that helps regulate blood sugar.

Insulin, Glucose, and Magnesium. Magnesium-rich foods also help normalize the insulin-glucose mechanism in the body. In at-the-table terms, this means more nuts, whole grains, leafy green vegetables, and beans.

Think Twice About Sweet or Salty. Refined sugars are rapidly absorbed into the bloodstream, causing a rise in blood sugar and in insulin, eventually exhausting the adrenals in a state of reactive hypoglycemia. Even if table sugar is out, garden sugar isn't. Stevia, a bush whose leaves are 330 times sweeter than cane sugar, can be bought in powder or liquid form or grown from seed. Fructose, used in moderation, is another sweetener that actually enhances sensitivity to insulin. But avoid products made with high-fructose corn syrup (HFCS), which contributes to metabolic syndrome, which in turn increases risk of diabetes and causes intra-abdominal fat, a risk factor for cardiovascular disease.

Herbs. Healing herbs, for taking in soups and juices, sprinkling on foods, or steeping as teas, that stimulate production of insulin include cinnamon, cloves, turmeric, bay leaf, fenugreek, and blueberry leaf.

Coffee and Tea. What you don't sip as juice, soup, or water, you can drink as coffee or tea. In a twelve-year study of more than 14,000 adults, women who drank three to four cups of coffee daily had a 20 percent reduced risk of diabetes type 2. The magic ingredient may be the antioxidant chlorogenic acid, which indirectly helps regulate blood glucose. But remember, caffeine is still problematic for other reasons, so check with your health care professional if you have a heart condition, ulcer, or another condition for which caffeine may be contraindicated. If you use decaf, make it organic to avoid the chemicals used to grow and process coffee beans.

Headaches

> Headaches affect the cardiovascular, nervous, and glandular immune centers.

There's Motrin and then there's minestrone when it comes to migraines or even a garden-variety headache. Whole foods that supply muscle relaxants like calcium, magnesium, and nerve-nourishing vitamin B₂ as well as EFAs can be both prescriptive and preemptive for cranial aches and pains.

What happens when your head aches? There is inflammation of the membranes lining the brain, the nerves of the cranium, and the upper neck, as well as dilation of blood vessels, with or without muscle spasms and with or without sinus congestion.

Behind the Pain

Headaches come in several varieties—cluster, tension (the commonest), simple and combination (tension headaches can trigger a migraine), and migraine, each originating in a different spot on the head—from the eyelids to the top and back of the skull. Ninety percent of us have had or will have tension headaches sooner or later (likelier for women than men). Causes are just as varied, so the first step is detecting the cause or triggers. Besides genetics, there is gender: 85 percent of adult migraine sufferers are female and 90 percent of all cluster headache victims are men (average age is twenty-eight to thirty). If you're female, falling estrogen levels can be the culprit.

Then there's stress, sleep disturbances, and food allergies, which are major factors in migraines, with many victims demonstrating sensitivity to one or more foods or to food additives such as the flavor enhancer MSG, the artificial sweetener aspartame, or the nitrite and sodium nitrate in luncheon meats and hot dogs. Tyramine is a substance found in caffeinated beverages, some cheeses, sour cream, red wine, and yes, despite its antioxidant content, chocolate. Tyramine increases blood flow to the brain in some people, causing headaches and migraines. Other foods that can affect blood pressure and precipitate headaches in the susceptible include cow's milk, citrus fruit, yeast products, dried fruit, and saturated fats, which contain arachidonic acid. Headaches can also be brought on by contraceptives or by overdoing alcohol and nicotine. A misaligned spine can create muscular tension in the cervical spine, which can progress, in a true head-bone-connected-to-anklebone fashion, into a chronic cranial ache. Migraines can even be triggered by falling or rising barometric pressure, as well as by heat, humidity, and even electrically charged dust particles.

What to Eat

Use soups formulated from whole organic or organically grown produce whenever possible, concentrating on fresh vegetables, rather than frozen or canned ones, and fruits that are sources of vitamin B complex, magnesium, calcium, vitamin D, and EFAs. Think (and shop) onions, garlic, soybeans, sesame, whole grains, and dairy or nondairy yogurt, plus cold-pressed oils, including olive and flaxseed. Eat regularly—preferably six small meals, avoiding caffeine and sugar.

And when you break for tea, before, during, or after that next headache, make it ginger, which decreases production of pain-producing prostaglandins. The substance called gingerol, which it secretes, is often as effective as aspirin in reducing inflammation.

Cancer

Cancer affects all six immune centers.

Think indole-3-carbinol (I3C) to sidestep or help heal from cancer. In nature, I3C is a cancer-blocking constituent of cruciferous vegetables (cabbage, broccoli, cauliflower, kale, bok choy, brussels sprouts) and may speed up the detoxification of many potentially toxic, tumor-promoting chemicals and also block the production of hormones linked to reproductive cancer.

Your soup spoon or salad fork can be valuable tools in the prevention and reversal of cancer—we need all the help we can get. According to the Environmental Working Group, the average American carries a body burden of ninety-plus industrial chemical pollutants, heavy metals, PCBs, and insecticides. Up to 10 percent of women carry mercury concentrations at levels that endanger the neurological health of a newborn. Worse, more than 3,000 chemicals are added regularly to our food supply and 1,000 new chemicals are introduced each year—many poorly tested or not tested at all.

Big C, Little C

In simple terms, cancer, which now affects one of every three women in North America, develops when changes to DNA (nucleic acids that are the basis of heredity, containing the genetic blueprint) produce malignant cells that replicate but are not controlled or killed by natural defense mechanisms in the body. Cancers can be hereditary, but to fully develop, there needs to be an environmental trigger. Indeed, according to the Columbia University Mailman School of Public

Health, 95 percent of cancers are caused by diet and environment, not by genes. For example, free radicals are created as the result of an oxidative process triggered by chemical toxins and unhealthy fats in the diet. Exposure to viruses, industrial pollutants, and radiation figure in, too.

In the case of radiation, no exposure is too small to initiate cellular damage, according to Dr. John W. Gofman, M.D., professor emeritus of molecular and cell biology at the University of California at Berkeley. Dr. Gofman's research finds that no amount of radiation, no matter how small it might be, is safe. He adds that exposure to radiation from medical procedures is a "highly important (probably the principal) cause of cancer and ischemic heart disease in America." Whole body scans, heart scans, PET scans, and virtual colonoscopies also emit tremendous amounts of radiation and should not be used for routine screening. Even magnetic resonance imaging scans (MRIs) and magnetic resonance angiograms (MRAs) emit electromagnetic radiations. Ultrasounds are completely safe. The cumulative effect from various sources of cancer-causing substances may take from five to thirty years to develop into actual tumors. Don't start counting, start eating and living according to precautionary principles. One day at a time may save your life.

What to Eat

Small changes for the better—like a big bowl of soup, especially when it's low fat—indeed pay big dividends. According to the National Cancer Institute (NCI), even a small reduction in daily fat intake—as little as 6 percent—can yield significant risk reduction. The NCI also recommends limiting salt, additives, animal products, and alcohol. The American Cancer Society agrees that 60 percent of cancer deaths could be prevented with a healthier lifestyle, including a cleaner diet. A daily dose of whole grains can boost the levels of your antioxidants that fight cancer. In fact, grains such as whole wheat, oats, and corn can have as many protective phytochemicals as fruits and vegetables, and sometimes more. According to Cornell University researchers, corn specifically has twice the antioxidant activity of whole wheat or brown rice. The soluble fiber found in grains and in raw produce helps prevent cancer by preventing the uptake of excess estrogen, a potential carcinogen.

The Stinking Rose Against a Stinking Disease. Regular consumption of garlic in salads, soups, sauces, and supplements has a significant effect on lowering cancer risk. In countries where large amounts of garlic and onion are consumed daily, stomach cancer risk is 90 percent lower than in countries where it is a sometimes thing. A study by researchers at the University of Texas M. D. Anderson Cancer Center suggests that four salads a week (as well as one or two low-impact exercise sessions) can help reduce your risk of lung cancer by 67 percent.

Try a Little Pineapple Salsa. According to researchers at the Queensland Institute of Medical Research in Australia, pineapple contains bromelain. An extract of crushed pineapple contains protease enzymes that block the growth of a broad range of tumor cells, including breast, lung, and colon. As a bonus, bromelain is a rich source of enzymes for digestion and reducing inflammation.

No to Pesticides and GMOs. Make that soup-or-salad-bowl produce organic to get more nutrients and avoid genetically modified organisms (GMOs). According to a University of California–Davis study, organically grown produce (which is also GMO-free) contained higher levels of natural cancer-fighting compounds than conventional samples. Antioxidant levels were as much as 50 to 60 percent higher than nonorganic.

Don't Forget to Use Your Bean. According to studies at the University of Missouri, soy protein may prevent and control both breast and colon cancers. Soy contains genistein, an isoflavone (plant estrogen) that helps halt the growth of breast cancer cells, sometimes by as much as 30 percent. Flaxseeds are another source of protective plant estrogens.

Nosh the Nutrient-Dense Plant Foods. Calcium-rich foods such as broccoli, citrus, leafy greens, and beans and the dishes that contain them are also protective. In a 2001 study of 800 women, those with the highest calcium intake had half the cancer rate of those with the least.

Bioflavonoids. Foods high in the bioflavonoid quercetin (apples, onions, grapefruit) are especially protective, as are lycopene- and carotene-rich fruits and vegetables such as citrus, cantaloupe, and carrots. Sweet potatoes (related to the morning glory) supply an average of 15,000 IU of vitamin A per potato. In one Hawaiian study, those who consumed the foods highest in quercetin were 40 to 50 percent less likely to develop lung cancer. As a bonus, the skins of foods such as apples and tomatoes contain cancer-fighting phenols, while the zest of citrus contains anticancer limonene. Juice the whole fruit or vegetable to benefit. Other foods with anticancer activity include carrots, tomatoes, cauliflower, asparagus, dandelion greens, spinach, kale, and almonds.

Eat More Omega-3s. The American Institute for Cancer Research also advises adding more inflammation-fighting omega-3 oils (olive oil, flax, salmon, grape seed, hemp, and walnuts and walnut oil) to your meal plans and cutting back on omega-6s (safflower, corn, soy, and peanut oils), which in large amounts appear to actually promote the disease.

Berries and More Berries. Keep the fruit bowl filled with more than citrus. Berries, because of the anthocyanins they contain, can reduce the risk of cancer, stroke, and heart disease and elevate LDL cholesterol. Anthocyanins act as free-radical scavengers in the body. Studies suggest that berries, especially red raspberries but also blackberries and strawberries, also provide ellagic acid, which enhances the antioxidant systems in the body and inhibits the initiation of tumors.

Drink Up! Water and high-water-content foods such as soups, juices, and watermelon do anticancer duty, too. Drinking filtered water can dilute potential carcinogens in the gastrointestinal tract and help prevent both stomach and colon cancer. Green tea, according to Japanese researchers, is rich in antioxidants and anti-inflammatory properties, which decrease the risk of seven different cancers and even block the early stages of colon cancer.

One and Two Make Four. To double your protection? Combine healing nutrients, as in soup making. For example, researchers in another study found that mushrooms rich in selenium give you thirteen times more protection when combined with cancer-fighting I3C-rich broccoli, than when the food was eaten separately.

Heart Disease

Heart disease affects all six immune centers.

Wherever you go, go with your whole heart, advised Confucius. The best place to take that whole heart these days would be the dinner table, if you need immune support.

Chicken soup (with or without the chicken) is not only good for the soul, it's pretty good therapy for the heart—in fact, for the whole cardiovascular system. That bisque, chowder, or consommé is triply therapeutic if you add cardio-protective herbs such as cayenne, garlic, or baby greens. The right foods can play a major part in keeping your cardio immune center (heart, lungs, and blood vessels) well and then some. And it can't be a half-hearted effort.

Have a Heart, Not a Heart Disease

One out of every fifty-eight Americans, or seventeen out of every thousand, says the National Health Institute, has atherosclerosis. More than 1.2 million of us suffer from cardiovascular disease (CVD), which covers a broad spectrum of disorders, including stroke, congestive heart failure, and birth defects of the heart and blood vessels. Heart attacks and strokes account for at least 40 percent of deaths from all causes, making CVD the number one killer each year. The incidence of death from heart attack is rising even among younger people ages 18 to 34. Many factors contribute, including high blood pressure, high bad cholesterol, elevated triglycerides, low good HDL cholesterol, smoking, diabetes, obesity, and a sedentary lifestyle. Other artery-damaging factors include high levels of glucose, iron, homocysteine, and fibrinogen and nonoptimal levels of C-reactive protein (CRP).

A smoothly functioning cardiovascular system is the result of good genes (having one parent with early heart disease doubles your own risk of cardio dysfunction), a targeted diet, exercise, weight in the normal range, and stress control. Stress may even top the list. A constant outpouring of stress hormones sets you up for heart disease like nothing else, cautions the American Heart Association, since these hormones release inflammatory chemicals, which allow LDL (bad) cholesterol to seep into arteries and stay there.

What to Eat

After all those fight-or-flight triggers, there's food—the good, the bad, and the in-between. A heart-smart diet if you're smart should contain plenty of low-fat vegetables and be rich in fiber, such as fruits, grains, and legumes. For add-on value, have a few nuts on the side—especially walnuts, which according to the ADA are helpful in preventing heart disease (therapeutic dose is one to two ounces daily). This is because the walnut appears to have a lower level of CRP, a marker for inflammation in the body. According to recent studies, traditional Mediterranean and Asian diets that are rich in nuts are associated with comparatively low rates of cardiovascular disease. Regular nut consumption may decrease the risk of heart disease by up to 50 percent. All nuts provide good fats, but walnuts provide alpha-linoleic as well as alpha-linolenic acids, along with the amino acid arginine, the B vitamin folic acid, fiber, and gamma-tocopherol (vitamin E), so their cardio-protective qualities include increased nitric acid formation, inhibited platelet aggregation, and decreased homocysteine levels.

Heart-boosting, cholesterol-lowering ingredients for the salad plate, soup bowl, and skillet include (but are not limited to):

▶ Extra-virgin olive oil provides abundant phenolic antioxidant compounds.

▶ Fish oils, flaxseed oil, and hemp seed oils provide omega-3 oils.

▶ Ginger is rich in compounds that relax the muscles surrounding the blood vessels and improve circulation.

▶ Turmeric, the spice that gives curry its color, has been shown to reduce blood vessel inflammation. In place of the spice itself, take a capsule of curcumin, the active ingredient in turmeric. The therapeutic daily dose is 400 to 600 milligrams.

▶ Garlic reduces the clotting tendency of the blood, helping to protect against strokes and heart attacks. (But it is contraindicated if you are on an aspirin or anticoagulant, such as warfarin, etc.) Even better, aged garlic extract (AGE), sold as a supplement, lowers total cholesterol, raises HDL, thins the blood, and lowers blood pressure—amazing benefits for an inexpensive, unassuming, ubiquitously useful everyday food.

Less Sodium, More Immunity. Shoot for 2,500 milligrams (less is even better) of sodium daily from meals, soup bowl, and shaker, keeping a sharp eye out for unlikely sources. It is not just in chips but also in vegetable juice cocktail (540 mg per 8-ounce glass) and rice pilaf mix (as much as 700 mg per 1 cup serving). In the susceptible, sodium can raise blood pressure and damage the heart and kidneys at high levels.

Baby Your Heart with Spinach. Besides watching sodium, upping potassium is critical, so pencil in a bowl of cream of spinach soup weekly and keep baby spinach around for quick salads. According to researchers at Johns Hopkins University in Baltimore, adding another

2,340 milligrams of this companion mineral to sodium to your diet (if your daily diet's supplying no more than the average 2,500 mg) may help you lower your blood pressure by as much as 25 percent, even preventing hypertension in the first place. Good sources of potassium (which also helps prevent stroke) include orange juice, raisins, cantaloupe, baked potatoes, and sea vegetables. It's thought that potassium (like diuretics) dilates blood vessels, causing them to relax. A pomegranate juice cocktail can also reduce plaque in the arteries, if it's there, by up to 33 percent. A few near beers can also help lower this plaque, say Spanish researchers (hops is the therapeutic ingredient, not alcohol).

The Peanut Butter Effect. Think nuts, legumes, and grains. Nonhydrogenated peanut butter is a good source of vitamin E, and a spoonful a day can also help keep cholesterol low. (Ditto raw almonds: a handful a day, unsalted and raw.) Look for brands enhanced with omega-3 oils. Spread it on soy or oat bread or whole-grain crackers, and you have a triple threat cardio snack. Oats provide fiber and vitamin B_6, which reduces homocysteine levels. Oatmeal is good, but oat bran is even better, providing twice the beta-glucan of oatmeal for lowering cholesterol 10 to 15 percent, providing roughage and stabilizing blood sugar.

Soy Immunity. Soy as a food or a "milk" provides isoflavones, which lower both total cholesterol and LDL and increase HDL. Aim for 30 to 60 milligrams of this compound daily from soy protein powders or soy foods.

Fruit Cocktail, Not Coronary Events. Fruit is your heart-healthy friend, too. A couple of kiwis a day can help lower your triglycerides by as much as 15 percent, as well as reducing platelet stickiness, according to Norwegian researchers. The fuzzy plum-sized New Zealand fruit also provides vitamin C and even vitamin E. Or take watermelon to heart. This juicy red fruit provides the amino acid citrulline, which protects against stroke, helps you heal from injuries, and lowers blood pressure.

Have a "big Mac" that's heart healthy. The pectin fiber in two apples (any variety) a day or twelve ounces of apple juice (or apple consommé) appears to keep bad LDL cholesterol from sticking to artery walls and damaging the cardio system. An improved blood profile can appear after only six weeks (no points for a high-fat, high-carb apple pie), say researchers at University of California–Davis.

Berries also belong on the cardio-protective menu. Reports from researchers at the U.S. Department of Agriculture in Oxford, Mississippi, indicate that blueberries in particular contain a compound called pterostilbene, which even in small doses appears to have the ability to lower cholesterol as effectively as some heart drugs by activating a cell receptor that helps lower blood fats, including cholesterol. The blueberry is also a richer source of antioxidants than thirty-nine other common fruits and vegetables.

Healthy Decadence. Dark chocolate also delays the body's absorption of LDL by as much as 8 percent, say researchers at Penn State University, while some Italian studies indicate dark chocolate boosts blood antioxidant levels by as much as 20 percent. Half an ounce a day is the therapeutic dose. But keep it dark: adding milk to chocolate cancels the antioxidant benefits. Also, chocolate contains satiric acid, a unique saturated fat that does not elevate cholesterol levels the way other saturated fats do. Dark chocolate also provides flavonoids that improve the functioning of the endothelial cells in the arteries.

Small Meals and Sterol-Supplemented Spreads. The tocotrienols found in rice bran, palm oil, and vitamin E–tocotrienol supplements also appear to affect cholesterol metabolism in a way similar to statin drugs. Snacking on six meals a day has a favorable effect on cholesterol. When you do give in to the bread-and-butter urge, use a butter substitute that contains cholesterol-lowering plant-based sterol esters (found in small amounts in fruits, vegetables, and whole grains), which can lower LDL by as much as 13 percent.

And don't neglect a daily glass of soy milk and an occasional glass of red wine. The latter is rich in cholesterol-blocking phytochemicals called saponins. Or bottoms up with grape juice, which provides compounds called flavonoids, which reduce blood-clotting tendencies (also found in apples and onions). Grapes also provide resveratrol, which inhibit cancer growth.

Soup Up, Blood Pressure Down. One of the best defenses to lower blood pressure is a mug of vegetarian vegetable soup a few times a week, with a little whole-grain bread on the side or sprouts on top. Blood pressure regulators from the garden include celery, garlic, tomatoes, and broccoli (or, better, broccoli sprouts). Broccoli delivers sulforaphane glucosinolate (SGS), which activates the body's natural detoxification system and antioxidant enzymes, helping protect the body from hypertension, atherosclerosis, and elevated cholesterol. Broccoli sprouts are even higher in SGS.

Beans and grains provide heart- and bowl-healthy fiber, as well as fiber that lowers CRP, elevated levels of which can lead to atherosclerosis. A high-fiber habit (aim for 30 to 35 g daily) may reduce your risk or a cardio crisis by as much as 50 percent. A study from the *Annals of Internal Medicine* analyzing data from studies of more than 300,000 participants concluded that for every 10 grams of fiber consumed there is a 14 percent reduction for all coronary events and a 27 percent reduction in coronary deaths.

Cardio-Protective Tomatoes. Tomatoes in your bowl or on your plate give you hypertension-placating lycopene (also found in grapefruit, watermelon, and apricots). Tomatoes also supply vitamin K, which protects the skeleton and keeps the blood-clotting function normal.

Celery and Edamame. Don't forget high-fiber celery. Recent lab tests suggest that celery may help decrease your total cholesterol, decrease your LDL (bad) cholesterol, and lower your blood pressure, something traditional Chinese medicine has always known. Top that celery with a sprinkle of ground flaxseed, which lowers LDL cholesterol (keep a shaker in the fridge). Another good fiber-rich, cholesterol-lowering snack to replace chips are unsalted, blanched edamame (soybeans) with a nutty, sweet flavor that is rich in protein.

A Slice of All-Star Pumpkin Pie. A little pumpkin (steamed, baked, or stewed) in your diet wouldn't hurt. Although they are grown in six of the seven continents, they aren't represented in six out of seven of our diets. But they should be, since they supply all-star heart-health nutrients, including zinc, omega-3s, vitamin E, folate, and magnesium.

Tea. That super immunity meal that gets you better gets even better if you wash it down with an occasional cup of hawthorn, linden, or yarrow tea. Three cups a day of these therapeutic tisanes can help lower blood pressure and relieve stress. (Stress leads to elevated blood pressure.) Ditto hibiscus, which is tasty hot or iced. To make a tea blend, combine 3 tablespoons each of loose leaves and use 1 teaspoon of the combo daily to brew a healing cup. Don't like tea? Make your own elixir, using liquid forms of all three herbs.

What Not to Eat: Foods to Subtract

Heart-hazardous ingredients include trans fats. Processed foods like microwave popcorn, instant noodles, processed cheeses, and even some low-fat milks have trans fats, which can clog arteries and lead to stroke and heart attacks. Trans fats boost LDL, lower HDL, and can triple your risk of a heart attack. Until recently, Americans were averaging 5.8 grams daily. Not healthy. Get to zero.

Controlling carbs and calories is also heart insurance. According to a 2004 National Academy of Sciences report, consistently eating an 1,100- to 1,950-calorie diet made up of 26 percent protein, 28 percent fat, and 46 percent carbohydrate can produce the vascular health of a twenty-year-old.

Insomnia

Insomnia affects the nervous, glandular, musculoskeletal, and respiratory immune centers.

Don't toss and turn—simmer and sip. Forty million of us, including 30 percent of seniors, don't get forty winks regularly. That's bad; failure to get a full night' sleep for a period of a month constitutes chronic insomnia. A majority are women, who are twice as likely to have difficulty sleeping as men, and it's even worse for postmenopausal women whose hormones keep them awake. If you're wide-eyed and wired when you should be winding down, sipping soup or tea can help.

Why White Nights?

Those "white nghts" (what the French call insomnia) that put you in a black or blue mood can have many causes, starting with cortisol imbalance (your levels of this hormone should be low, not on high alert) caused by inflammation somewhere in the body, which in turn depresses DHEA and causes sleeplessness. Have both hormone levels tested to be sure. Other causes include stress and all-American anxiety, depression, poor diet, excess caffeine, food allergies, and a number of medications whose side effects include disturbed sleep, or any combination of these. Of course, simply being middle-aged means you sleep less and sleep less well. Menopause also disrupts sleep patterns—and that's not good. Full insomnia leads to a reduced ability to process information, slowed reaction time, reduced creativity, and increased risk of accidents.

Americans (who get less than the therapeutic seven hours a night of sleep) spend more than $2 billion on prescribed sleep inducers with all of their attendant risks. Sleep deprivation is no small dysfunction, since the body conducts most of its repair functions nocturnally. Worn or damaged cells that go unrepaired can lead to pain and illness. Poor sleep patterns even affect the health of your connective tissue, which is repaired during sleep. Poor healing may lead to joint instability, according to the National Institute of Chiropractic Research. Short-form snoozing may lead to weight gain. Studies show that getting only four or five hours of sleep nightly increases your risk of being overweight or obese by more than 50 to 70 percent, since it decreases the levels of a natural appetite-suppressing hormone and increases levels of an appetite-stimulating hormone. It also lowers testosterone levels in men, reduces immunity, and may even increase the risk for coronary heart disease and high blood pressure, says the American Council on Collaborative Medicine. Inadequate sleep also ages us by depriving bodies of oxygen, elevating blood pressure, and increasing levels of stress hormones. As well, it can weaken the immune system and increase the risk of high blood pressure and heart disease.

What to Eat

The Fluids Rx. Fortunately, there are ways to get that shut-eye, starting with soup, juice, and tea. The best soup-bowl ingredients for regulating sleep-inducing hormones include fresh fruits, especially bananas, figs, and dates; fresh vegetables, especially lettuce and the juices of carrots, celery, and spinach; whole grains and nuts, especially cashews, almonds, and walnuts; low-fat dairy products, including yogurt; and foods or ingredients rich in neuromuscular nutrients (calcium and magnesium), such as yogurt and kefir. Sleepy-time teas include catnip, chamomile, kava kava, passion flower, and hops.

Indigestion

Indigestion affects the nervous, glandular, and digestive/detoxification immune centers.

"I stand in awe of my body," said Thoreau. You should, too—especially your gut. More than 60 percent of the body's antibodies are produced there.

The gastrointestinal tract, all twenty feet or so of it, is the seat of the greater immune system and the heart of the digestive immune center. An awesome lot can go wrong there—and does. As many as 40 percent of all Americans experience heartburn or some related symptom once a month and some 10 percent do so daily, according to the American Society of Gastroenterology. Other troubles like flatulence, diarrhea, constipation, diverticulitis, peptic ulcer, malabsorption syndrome, and irritable bowel syndrome (IBS), which may afflict up to 30 percent of the population, aren't far behind. Although we reach for antacids (six million of us take them to mask the gut distress caused by arthritis meds alone), over-the-counter and prescription drugs that can irritate and often damage the stomach lining aren't the answer. Eating the right foods in the right combinations and in the right amounts, as well as avoiding the troublemakers, could be.

Tract Tactics

Is it any wonder that your stomach needs a little roadside assistance now and then? The normal digestive tract is home to some ten quarts of digestive juices produced daily by the stomach, pancreas, liver, and intestinal wall. The not-so-normal gastrointestinal tract may come up short (especially if it is deficient in vitamin B$_6$ or zinc). Gradually increasing your intake of enzyme-rich raw foods such as apples, bananas, grapes, pineapple, carrots, and celery will help normalize gut function. So will the use of digestive enzymes with each meal (especially if you are over forty, which is when digestive juice production slows). Combining foods properly is another restorative strategy, particularly avoiding the combination of starches and proteins (especially animal proteins) in the same meal.

Of course, your digestive dysfunction may go beyond the garden-variety gastrointestinal complaints. What seems like IBS may actually be LGS (leaky gut syndrome), the culprit behind a range of autoimmune diseases such as rheumatoid arthritis and fibromyalgia, says Dr. Leo Galland of the Foundation for Integrated Medicine. Look for a holistic physician who can administer the lactulose/mannitol challenge to find out. Long-term use of NSAIDS (nonsteroidal anti-inflammatory drugs) such as Advil, steroids like cortisone and pred-

nisone, and antibiotics contribute by killing off friendly bacteria in
the gut and creating a breeding ground for parasites, yeast, and, in
turn, LGS.

When Indigestion Is Something More

Also consider the possibility that the problem may be grains, not the
gut. A small percentage of sufferers with IBS-like symptoms are actually suffering from celiac disease (CD), which is an allergy to gluten.
Gluten is the protein in grains such as wheat, rye, barley, spelt, and
triticale, and even small exposures can cause bloating, diarrhea, and
fatigue. Untreated, it can lead to malnutrition and osteoporosis.

Fructose intolerance and fructose malabsorption (which affects
30 to 50 percent of the population) are conditions in which the small
intestine cannot absorb the sugar in fruit, processed foods, and juices.
These conditions can cause bloating, cramping, and flatulence syndrome, as well as trigger mood swings and sugar cravings. Avoid soft
drinks and processed juices, and eating fruit only in moderation is
remedial.

Too Little Acid, Not Too Much?

Last but not at all least, your stomach could be secreting too *little* acid
rather than too much—known as hypochlorhydria, or insufficient
hydrochloric acid (HCl). By age forty, 40 percent of us are affected,
and by age fifty, it's 50 percent. If your symptoms improve after taking
betaine HCl available as a supplement, you have your solution.

If you have no stomach complaints and want to keep it that way—
eat small meals, not big; eat in stress-free surroundings; and avoid
foods that you're allergic to or intolerant of (the short list includes
wheat, dairy, eggs, citrus, and soy).

What to Eat

Consider the following twelve ways to keep that 20-foot tract intact.

1. Learn the lesson of less. Consider what you might subtract from your three square meals. For starters, eliminate refined sugar, refined grains, highly processed foods, carbonated drinks, all foods that become acid in the system—including meat and shellfish, dairy foods, as well as artificial sweeteners, coffee, and alcoholic drinks.

2. Avoid the GERD triggers, and up the fiber. Gastroesophageal reflux disease (GERD) may be turned on by white bread, chocolate, tomatoes, tomato sauce, and citrus. Eat around those, and instead get 25 to 30 grams of fiber a day from fruits, vegetables, and grains, which can reduce your risk of heartburn by as much as 20 percent. IBS sufferers need 25 to 40 grams of soluble fiber with plenty of water.

The following chart shows what hikes gut immunity best.

Ten Top Sources of Fiber

FOOD	SERVING	GRAMS
Barley, cooked	½ cup	13
Raspberries	1 cup	8
Wheat bran	½ cup	8.4
Flaxseed meal	¼ cup	8
Kidney beans	½ cup	8
Carrot, raw	2 large	8
Almonds	½ cup	8
Spinach	2 cups cooked	8
Winter squash	1 cup cooked	6
Figs	3 dried	5–6

Note: It's important to get a combination of both soluble and insoluble fibers in the daily diet. Fruits, vegetables, and oats provide soluble fiber, while whole grains, bran, and legumes (as well as some fruits and vegetables) are sources of insoluble fiber.

3. Cut salt intake and stop smoking. Both habits encourage acid reflux.

4. Up your garlic and onion (if you tolerate them). All members of the *Allium cepa* family promote digestion and encourage the release of toxins from the gastrointestinal tract. (Note they are a source of flatulence for some.)

5. The other O. Shift the balance from omega-6 oils such as corn, sunflower, and safflower so prevalent in the standard American diet to inflammation-fighting oils such as flax, hemp, grape seed, olive, and canola. Look for an organic blend of at least two to benefit more.

6. Hydrate with dandelion root tea. Three cups a day can ease IBS symptoms (as well as allergy symptoms). Dandelion stimulates the growth of good bacteria in the gut. Try ginger soup or peppermint tea as a better response to GERD and other garden-variety digestive complaints than any commercial antacid.

7. Consider herbal bitters for relieving heartburn, indigestion, and even low stomach acid. Bitters are liquid herbal combinations that include botanicals such as dandelion, gentian, yarrow, devil's claw, and bitter orange.

8. Peppermint oil. The German Commission E, a government regulatory agency composed of scientists, physicians, pharmacists, and toxicologists who evaluate the usefulness and safety of herbs, recommends enteric-coated tablets of peppermint oil (one capsule three times daily) for diarrhea and constipation, as well as bloating and cramps. After you get over your symptoms, take a good whiff of peppermint to run faster. Studies from the Wheeling Jesuit University in West Virginia indicate that as an aromatherapy scent, peppermint increases activity in the wake-up center of the brain.

9. Go green. Asian studies indicate that gastritis and stomach cancer rates are only half as high among dedicated green tea sippers. Look for an organic brand containing a standardized extract.

10. Avoid antacids. These can drop stomach acid levels too low, causing excessive acid levels with extended use or leading to bleeding in the gastrointestinal tract. In any case, the aluminum that acid-blockers may contain is unhealthy. Use artichoke leaf extract to ease that sense of fullness and bloating. Artichoke leaf extract even helps lower cholesterol, advises the Herbal Research Foundation. Try 1 teaspoon three times daily. Or reach for the teapot and brew chamomile tea, which is widely used throughout Europe for digestive ills, including inflammation of the intestinal tract. Ditto ginger tea, which is used as an inflammatory and is also good for travel sickness and nausea.

11. Avoid processed foods containing trans fats, which are linked not only to heart disease but also to GERD and heartburn.

12. Taste your way to better digestive health. According to the Ayurvedic concept of the six tastes, including one of each of the following tastes—pungent, astringent, sweet, sour, salty, and bitter—in each meal leads to a balanced diet through the sense of taste, which translates into improved digestion. If you are susceptible to heartburn, watch out for foods that can trigger it—especially chocolate, tea, coffee, fatty foods, spices, citrus, sugar, and tomatoes.

Osteoporosis

> Osteoporosis affects the glandular and musculoskeletal immune centers.

Bad bones are bad news. More than 44 million of us over the age of fifty have them in the form of osteoporosis or as the low-bone-mass syndrome (often a precursor to osteoporosis) called osteopenia. Both signal a loss of calcium from the bones, occurring most frequently in postmenopausal women and men over seventy. Symptoms, if there are any, include low back pain, stooped posture, loss of height, and increased risk of fracture.

According to a 2003 study in the *British Medical Journal*, breaking your leg at age sixty-five or older increases your risk of death twelve times over, and of the 1.5 fractures annually, 50 percent are spinal and 50 percent are hips and wrists. If you are among the vulnerable, the odds of a fracture are one in three—not good odds.

Good Defenses, Good Bones

Conversely, strong bones mean a strong immune system, and the reverse is also true. Chronic inflammatory conditions such as rheumatoid arthritis are related to a higher osteoporosis risk, and even minor immune system malfunctions can affect bones by increasing the activity of cells that break down bones.

Your knee bone is connected to your anklebone, and your anklebone is connected to your heart muscle, in a sense. Osteoporosis and homocysteine, for example, also go together. Higher levels of this substance, which is linked—like cholesterol and triglycerides—to heart disease, can double your risk of fractures as well, say researchers.

Women Are at Higher Risk

Thinning bones are a bigger red flag than cancer, at least for women. According to the National Osteoporosis Foundation, a woman's risk of hip fracture, the most dangerous result of osteoporosis, is equal to the risk of breast, ovarian, and uterine cancers combined. While after the age of thirty calcium is no longer busy building bone, dietary calcium is still critical. There are five risk factors you can't change, including age, gender, and family history, but you *can* change seven, including smoking (don't do it), alcohol (be moderate), and diet.

What to Eat

The ten top fruits, vegetables, and grains for getting the vitamins, minerals, and trace elements that partner to keep you tough and tall include whole grains such as oats; fresh fruits such as peaches, citrus, berries, pineapple, and grapes; fresh vegetables such as tomatoes, carrots, and broccoli; leafy greens such as collard, kale, mustard, dandelion greens, and parsley; and soy foods.

Tomatoes and Flaxseed: Pair Them for Bone Benefits. According to studies at the University of Toronto in Canada, lycopene, the star antioxidant in tomatoes, stimulates the activity of bone-forming cells, or osteoblasts, while inhibiting mineral resorption. (It also reduces fibroids and helps keep the prostate healthy.) A 2004 study at Oklahoma State University revealed that diets that included a daily dose of flaxseeds or flax caused a decrease in bone resorption and calcium loss.

Check Your Fatty Acid Intake. Bones need essential fatty acids (EFAs) to flourish, especially those EFAs (omega-3 and omega-6 oils) found in oils such as grape seed, olive, flax, hemp, and wheat germ. The omega-3 fatty acids in some of these oils, for example, suppress production of cytokines, compounds that stimulate skeletal breakdown. Some studies indicate that omega-3s (also found in fish oils) are especially useful in preventing osteoporosis of the hip and spine. But don't overdo that salad dressing or soup drizzle. Excess oils have the opposite effect of inhibiting the uptake of calcium from the gastrointestinal tract.

Get Your Vitamins A and C. Vitamin A and Vitamin C foods are needed to manufacture protein in the bones. You get them both in dark leafy greens, cantaloupe, tomatoes, and peppers. This may be as important as calcium for preventing age-related fractures.

Vitamin K. Vitamin K serves as a biological glue that attaches calcium to the bone matrix and helps produce a specific protein found in bone tissue. This process occurs naturally in your intestines, so eat those dark leafy greens and cabbage family vegetables like brussels sprouts and bok choy to get more.

Potassium. You need this mineral to buffer acid in the body. You can get it from Swiss chard, spinach, winter squash, and soybeans.

Vegan Bones. Make bone building easier by becoming a vegan. Because diets rich in animal protein cause the body to lose calcium, by going vegan, you need less calcium to stay in calcium balance. It's smarter to get your edible calcium from broccoli, beans, nuts, dried fruits, soy and rice milks, sprouts, and vegetables. Did you know that 2 ounces of sea vegetables, such as arame, kelp, and hijiki, contain as much calcium as half a can of sardines—without the ocean pollutants and with a wider range of trace minerals for skeletal well-being?

Put on the Tea. The flavonoid antioxidants in black tea appear to stimulate production of new cells that build bone. In an Australian study of 1,500 older women, regular tea drinkers had higher hip-bone density than those who abstained. If you're avoiding caffeine, decaf does the trick, too.

Bad for Bones, Especially for Bad Bones

Bread and Bones Often Go Together. Twenty-five percent of people with untreated celiac disease (an inherited intestinal disorder in which the body cannot absorb gluten) have brittle bones. In those suffering from this disease, consumption of gluten damages the lining of the intestine, preventing the uptake of calcium and leaching the bones of alkaline minerals such as calcium and magnesium. A healthy diet causes the diet to be more alkaline than acid and includes vegetables and fruit (such as citrus, which is acid in nature but alkaline-producing in the body. Ditto balsamic vinegar.) But hold the acid-producing meat and dairy.

Get Your D. As many as 60 percent of us are D-deficient. Vitamin D (which is really a hormone) may increase calcium absorption in the gastrointestinal tract by up to 65 percent. Vitamin D also decreases excretion by the kidneys. According to the American Medical Association, it even improves muscle strength in older adults. To trigger its production in your skin, spend fifteen minutes in the sun—without sunblock, which inhibits vitamin D. As a bonus, cholecalciferol (vitamin D_3) also helps ward off colon and breast cancer and protects against hypertension.

Get the Right Amount of Protein. Protein builds bones, but too much can cause calcium loss, which in turn can cause bone loss. Are you getting too little or too much? Thirty to forty percent of men and women over age 70 fall below the DV for protein, but the typical midlife American woman eats 50 percent more than she needs, says the Women's Health Project. Protein should account for only 20 percent of the calories you take in. Does it? Check it out.

Got Milk or Not Milk? Milk (and more calcium) may not be the osteo-building answer, especially if that milkshake is part of a high-protein diet. According to a WHO report, hip fracture rates are higher in countries where dairy consumption is high. The Nurses' Health Study indicates that neither milk nor calcium reduced fracture rates better than vitamin D intake from foods and supplements did.

Avoid Certain Drugs. Bone remodeling and regeneration continue twenty-four hours a day, creating an entirely new skeleton every eight years. But you can slow that down if you use immunosuppressive drugs like steroids, which cause bone loss. Be careful of SSRI drugs, too. So-called selective serotonin reuptake inhibitors put you at a higher risk of hip bone loss, according to a five-year study with more than 2,000 older women with thinning bones. A similar larger study with older men produced similar results.

Calcium Dos and Don'ts List

It is estimated that more than 70,000 hip fractures could be prevented yearly if adults older than age sixty-five who currently don't take calcium and vitamin D started supplementing. It matters even more as we age, since calcium is also important for the health of the heart, blood pressure, and the menstrual cycle.

▶ Do take the right form. Calcium is poorly absorbed, so get it from better-absorbed forms such as calcium citrate, lactate, or an aspartate form. But avoid carbonate, which can cause digestive upsets if the stomach acid level is low. Take it in divided doses to improve absorption. If you take the bone-building mineral supplement strontium citrate, another natural bone builder, take it apart from calcium on an empty stomach.

▶ Fiber supplements can interfere with calcium absorption, so take them a few hours apart. This also applies to antibiotics, steroids, and thyroid medications.

▶ Take calcium separately from caffeine, alcohol, fructose, and animal protein when possible.

▶ Don't use antacids as calcium supplements. Stomach acid is critical to the absorption of this mineral.

Vision Disorders

Vision disorders affect the nervous and glandular immune centers.

Ninety-six percent of the universe is invisible to us, say cosmologists. And how well do we manage the 4 percent that's in plain view? Not so well, apparently. When the visionary immune center is running on nutritional near-empty, anything from dry eye syndrome (DES) to age-related macular degeneration (AMD) can and does result. More than a million Americans over age forty are blind, and millions more suffer from some sort of visual shortfall—nearsightedness, farsightedness, night blindness, presbyopia, dry eyes, and simply tired eyes. Worse, those numbers are expected to double over the next three decades, according to the National Eye Institute.

Consider AMD, which is the leading cause of blindness. Eight million of us older than age fifty-five are at serious risk for this disorder, which blurs the sharp central vision by destroying the macula of the eye. It is painless, and like glaucoma it can advance slowly with few clues that vision is deteriorating.

Glaucoma, which affects some 3 million Americans, is an imbalance in the production and drainage of fluid in the eye, which in turn causes a buildup of pressure that can damage the optic nerve. People over the age of sixty-five, the very nearsighted, African-Americans, people with diabetes, and hypertension victims are most at risk. If you have a genetic susceptibility, all you may need is some oxidative stress to activate it.

In cataracts, damage to the protein of the lens of the eye causes clouding, which impairs vision. This oxidation can occur as a result of smoking, exposure to the sun, and other environmental threats. Toxic levels of lead in the body can also contribute to cataract formation. Nothing is known to fully reverse the condition. Symptoms are blurred vision, seeing spots, or a sense of a film covering the eye.

Then there's night blindness: a difficulty with seeing well in dim or dark light is an indication of a deficiency of vitamin A, necessary for the production of visual purple.

What to Eat: Visionary Foods

The good news is that there are plenty of oh-say-can-you-see solutions within reach. Here are seven for starters:

1. Pick from vegetables rich in the various carotenoids found in carrots, collards, mustard greens, sweet potatoes, and spinach. It is said that the amount of lutein in half a cup of spinach, eaten regularly, may cut the risk of AMD in half. Lutein and zeaxanthin are the two carotenoids in the retina that are critical for good ocular function. The macula also contains a high concentration of carotenoids that protect against UV light and blue filter light, the primary sources of oxidative damage.

2. Focus on concentrated mixtures of foods that intensify nutrients such as

  ▷ multivegetable soups like minestrone and gazpacho
  ▷ multivegetable salads
  ▷ fruit smoothies with three to six ocular-nutrient-rich fruits
  ▷ fruit salads and dessert soups

3. Besides the usual bananas, apples, and berries, also include rhubarb, which is high in vitamin A, and kiwis, which supply more lutein than any other fruit or vegetable except corn. (A daily fuzzy fruit can also lower your potential for clots and reduce triglycerides.)

4. Don't forget berries, the number one best source of antioxidants. The purple pigment in bilberries and other dark berries called anthocyanins regenerate an essential protein in the eye called visual purple. Anthocyanins protect the eyes from free radical damage caused by age and sunlight. Get out of your berry comfort zone, and try the more exotic and more nutrient-dense goji berries or acai berries (which have twenty times more antioxidants than red wine). Both are available as a dried snack and as a supplement.

5. Other vision-strengthening nutrients include zinc, found in whole grains, beans, and nuts (as well as meat and poultry for nonvegetarians). Zinc is essential for the synthesis of the enzyme that controls retinal function.

6. Keep the following in your freezer, fridge, or cupboard:
   ▷ flaxseeds and chia seeds
   ▷ walnuts, Brazil nuts, and soybeans
   ▷ sea vegetables (and safe fish, if you eat it) for the omega-3 fatty acids, which fight ocular inflammation and reduce the risk of AMD and glaucoma. Experiment: try dulse crumbled on salads in place of bacon bits, hijiki steamed and tossed with pasta, kelp sprinkled on vegetables in place of salt and pepper, and arame in the vegetarian hash.

7. Drink up. Water and high-water foods such as lettuce and juicy fruits such as peaches, plums, and melon make everything in the body work better, especially dry and fatigued eyes.

YOUR SUPER IMMUNITY
PROGRAM

YOU CAN'T MAXIMIZE IMMUNITY without a program, and no program is complete without transformative recipes, meal plans, and tips to bond you to those foods that turn your health around one bean, berry, or leafy green at a time.

Super Immunity Recipes

Now that you know which twenty-five super immunity foods to get into your diet, here are almost one hundred super immunity recipes with more than two hundred variations that combine those foods in countless disease-busting, health-boosting ways, to empower all six of your body's immune centers, from breakfast to late-night snacks. For a total super immunity program, see the last section, starting on page 222, for easy meal plans that will help you supercharge your immunity in just four weeks.

Super Immunity Nutritional Tips

"One cannot think well, love well, sleep well, if one has not dined well," observed Virginia Woolf. It might be added one cannot dine well without dining on the right foods. Here's how to make the most of what comes out of your kitchen and goes into your mouth.

▶ **The power of two:** Before you splash into your first bowl of soup for the day, clean your system. Put the juice of two lemons in a small pitcher of water. Sip this throughout the day. Or get your immune-boosting antioxidants from two cups of (organic) green tea daily or two cups of Rooiboos (it's red, it's robust, it's South African high-powered nutritional bush).

▶ **Super cinnamon:** Keep a shaker of cinnamon table-ready. Add to fruit and other sweet soups, or dust croutons for fruit soups. Cinnamon contains antimicrobial compounds that inhibit bacteria and viruses. A half teaspoon of cinnamon daily (in or out of your soup bowl) helps the body use insulin more efficiently and cuts blood sugar levels by up to 30 percent.

▶ **Zest your way to a happier gut:** Keep that rind you peeled off your next orange, tangerine, or tangelo. It's a good source of probiotics, a kind of carbohydrate that feeds the good bacteria in your intestinal tract, helping prevent the growth of gastrointestinal pathogens. Use the zest atop spicy soups, in muffins, and with crackers.

▶ **Spoon up to maximize your vitamin E:** Taking your daily vitamin E supplement with your daily mug of minestrone or consommé ensures that you get your supplement's worth. Vitamin E is absorbed more efficiently and retained at higher levels, studies show, when taken with a meal-like soup, rather than without. Another key to better absorption: take natural vitamin E—look for d-tocopherol, rather than dl-tocopherol (synthetic) on the label.

▶ **A cupful of tea keeps the cardiologist away:** Studies show that regular consumption of black tea may reduce your risk of heart disease by half. The secret ingredient is catechins, a be-kind-to-your-cardio-system chemical found in all teas but especially in black varieties. Another way to capitalize on catechins: be on the watch for recipes where tea will work as well as the water that's called for.

▶ **Oil up for antioxidants:** For add-on antioxidants, add a few drops of cold-pressed vegetable or nut oil to your bowl before serving up. This increases your absorption of antioxidants, especially beta-carotene, which is poorly absorbed without fat.

▶ **Spice up for super immunity:** Keep a shaker of the curry spice turmeric next to the salt and pepper. Turmeric is more than a must for curry. It's preventive medicine with anticancer and anti-inflammatory properties. Add a dash to any soup that begs for a little bite.

▶ **Super immunity your garlic:** After chopping or mashing garlic, let it rest a few minutes—this pause is said to increase garlic's infection-fighting properties.

▶ **Strawberry is for C:** Did you know that one extra strawberry a day is what you need to get the extra 15 milligrams of vitamin C now recommended by the National Academy of Sciences? Of course, more is even better. Keep a bowl of tomato soup in the fridge to get a megadose of water-soluble C in each spoonful.

▶ **Zinc without meat:** Are you a tofu-totaler? Don't forget an occasional 30-milligram capsule of zinc, an important immune enhancer that vegetarians are often short on. But more isn't more. Amounts greater than 100 milligrams can actually depress immunity. Besides animal products where that zinc is accompanied by saturated fat, arachidonic acid, and traces of hormones and pesticides, zinc is found in whole grains, seeds, nuts, and vegetables like peas, mushrooms, and sea vegetables.

▶ **Block that buzz:** House blends at high-end coffee shops like Starbuck's have up to 50 percent more caffeine than other java stops. In fact, don't drink coffee or tea with that mineral-rich lunchtime soup. Both contain tannin, which reduces iron absorption by up to 94 percent. This includes some herbal teas like peppermint, which also interferes with iron uptake.

▶ **Do the flax grind:** Keep a pepper grinder on the table filled with flaxseeds to add extra omega-3s to meals (refrigerate between meals).

Super Immunity Culinary Tips

▶ Sautéing your dark greens in a calorie-insignificant amount of olive oil rather than steaming over water will provide five times as much of the antioxidant beta-carotene.
▶ Add a little fat (real butter, oil, an avocado) to your carotene-carrying fruits and vegetables (red, green, yellow, and orange) to absorb more vitamins A, E, and K. Fat acts as a nutrient transporter.
▶ Keep the dice small when cutting fruits, to keep oxidation to a minimum and preserve vitamin C.
▶ Instead of toast triangles, serve "quilts." Just put bread that has been battered for fresh toast into the waffle maker.
▶ Add coconut oil to the water when boiling rice. It coats the grains and adds trace amounts of beta-carotene, potassium, and mono-unsaturated fat.
▶ Keep your flour for dusting in a saltshaker. And use a wire whisk in place of a flour sifter.
▶ If you rinse the fresh parsley before it is ready to garnish, you lose that nice-to-the-nose aroma.
▶ Using raw vegetables in a cold soup? Cut the bitterness of broccoli, brussels sprouts, and broccoli raab by blanching in salt water one to three minutes before adding to the bowl.
▶ Avoiding or reducing salt? Use a splash of vinegar or lemon juice to give a hint of saltiness without the sodium. Or season with

kelp or dulse powder to get the nutrients you may be missing, such as iodine and vitamin B_{12}.

► Cut tomatoes for that tomato bisque with a serrated knife, which will slice without mashing flesh.

► Savor spicy? A dash of pepper vinegar in almost any soup is a pick-me-up, especially where there's no added salt.

► Vanilla and vegetables: a dash of vanilla (believe it or not) in spicy tomato or chili soups can cut acidity and add a charming mystery note.

► Add a few slices of fresh gingerroot to cooking water when preparing simple vegetable soups.

► To thicken any soup (without starch), puree cooked vegetables in a blender and return the puree to the soup pot.

► A little dry wine will add flavor to almost any soup. What else does?

▷ Try summer savory and cloves to flavor minestrone.

▷ Try thyme and cayenne pepper in milk-based soups.

▷ Use thyme and marjoram in vegetable combinations.

▷ A pinch of mustard enhances bean soups.

▷ One teaspoon vinegar can help enhance the flavor for each quart of vegetable soup. Or use vinegar plus a pinch of sugar in each quart of legume soup.

▷ For a little extra salt-free saltiness, add 1 teaspoon wine to the soup pot before serving.

▷ Use fresh-ground peppercorns in thick soups and chowders.

► Peel garlic cloves, and place in freezer bags. Frozen garlic is easy to chop and is odor-free while frozen.

► To speed-peel a large amount of garlic for any soup, brush whole heads with oil, place in a 400°F oven, and bake until the skin slips off easily, about ten to fifteen minutes.

► To turn any soup into a cream of soup, add a cup of dairy or nondairy milk and blend. Thicker yet? Add a cup of plain yogurt (after soup has cooled) or extra-soft tofu.

▶ Less is best when stir-frying vegetables for a soup. When heated, oil thins and disperses. A half teaspoon applied to a paper towel, for example, is enough to lubricate two baking sheets, and 1 tablespoon will coat 2 pounds of still-warm cooked potatoes.

▶ Store your fruits and vegetables in produce bags formulated to reduce ethylene gases and to slow spoilage and nutrient loss. Go to www.reusablebags.com for details, or ask at your local market.

Note: With the exception of dairy alternatives to soy or rice and an occasional egg, these recipes do not include animal products. It is certainly possible to substitute any meat, poultry, or fish for the plant-based central ingredients in many of the main dishes that follow. When you do, keep in mind that unless they are organic, these foods come with the burden of unhealthy saturated fats, growth hormones, chemical residues (meat and poultry), toxins like PCBs, and heavy metals (in many types of fish). Animals raised for food also for the first time in history are generating more greenhouse gases than trains, planes, and automobiles and are contributing mightily to both land and water degradation, according to the United Nations Food and Agriculture Organization (FAO). Every meatless meal you have can make a difference.

BREAKFAST

Cream of Quinoa and Cranberries

YIELD: 4 servings

PREPARATION TIME: 30 minutes

The complex carbs in quinoa will keep you energized, while the grain's high protein keeps you alert; also rich in good-for-the-heart lignans.

1½ cups vanilla soy milk, plus more for topping each serving

½ cup water

¼ teaspoon salt

1 cup quinoa, rinsed and drained

½ cup dried cranberries

2 tablespoons maple, date, or other raw natural sugar

1 teaspoon cinnamon

½ teaspoon ground ginger

¼ teaspoon allspice or ground cloves

½ cup chopped, toasted pecans (topping)

Bring soy milk, water, and salt to a boil. Stir in quinoa and cranberries. Reduce heat to medium-low, and simmer about 15 minutes, stirring occasionally until grains are tender and liquid is absorbed. Remove from heat, and stir in sugar and spices.

Serve warm, topped with more soy milk and nuts.

··· **VARIATIONS** ···

▶ Use low-fat dairy milk instead of soy.

▶ Use dried blueberries or goji berries in place of cranberries.

▶ Omit any of the spices.

▶ Use sunflower seeds in place of pecans.

Flaxberry Flapjacks

YIELD: 4 servings

PREPARATION TIME: 15 minutes

Flax for your bad cholesterol, berries for your brain, soy for your bones.

1½ cups unbleached all-purpose flour

2 tablespoons sugar or natural sweetener, to taste

2 teaspoons baking powder

½ teaspoon salt

2 tablespoons ground flaxseeds

¼ cup water

1¼ cups soy milk or other dairy-free milk

1 teaspoon vanilla extract

¼ cup fresh blueberries or frozen blueberries, thawed

In a large bowl, combine flour, sugar, baking powder, and salt, and set aside.

Combine ground flaxseeds and water in blender, and blend until thick, about half a minute (flax replaces eggs here). Add soy milk and vanilla, and process until smooth.

Pour the wet ingredients into the dry ingredients, mixing with a few rapid strokes until just moist. Fold in berries.

Preheat oven to 200°F. Heat a lightly oiled skillet over medium heat. Ladle about 3 tablespoons of batter onto the hot griddle. Cook flapjack on one side until small bubbles appear on top (about 2 minutes). Flip pancake with a metal spatula, and cook until the other side is lightly browned (about 1 minute more).

Keep cooked flapjacks warm in oven while preparing the remaining pancakes.

VARIATIONS

► Substitute fresh raspberries, strawberries, or a more exotic berry such as acai or goji.

► Use dairy milk instead of soy.

Black-and-Blue Syrup

YIELD: 1½ cups

PREPARATION TIME: 20 minutes

Tasty and immune-boosting spooned warm on pancakes,
waffles, or French toast or dribbled cold over yogurt.

2 cups fresh or frozen blueberries
½ cup fresh-squeezed orange juice
¼ teaspoon lemon juice, fresh-
   squeezed or bottled
1 tablespoon chopped fresh mint

2 tablespoons sugar or 1 teaspoon
   stevia, to taste
½ teaspoon cinnamon
2 tablespoons cornstarch dissolved
   in ¼ cup water

Combine all ingredients in a saucepan, and bring to a boil. Reduce heat
and cook, uncovered and stirring occasionally, until sauce thickens to the
consistency of maple syrup.

Spoon over pancakes, French toast, or waffles or serve cold over berries or yogurt.

··· VARIATIONS ···

► Use blackberries instead of blueberries.
► Use ¼ teaspoon mint extract in place of mint leaves.

Breakfast Bruschetta

YIELD: 6 servings

PREPARATION TIME: 1½ hours

Why two honeys? The mild spiciness of the clover honey amplifies the tang of the tomatoes roasting; later, the hearty buckwheat honey balances the creaminess of the cheese.

2 pints cherry or grape tomatoes, halved lengthwise

1½ tablespoons extra-virgin olive oil

2 tablespoons clover honey

2 teaspoons fresh thyme leaves or 1 teaspoon dried

1 teaspoon coarse salt

Pinch black pepper or kelp powder

12 baguette slices, ½ inch thick, cut diagonally

1 cup fresh ricotta, farmer's cheese, or crumbled tofu

2 tablespoons buckwheat honey

2 teaspoons fresh chopped basil or 1 teaspoon dried

Preheat oven to 300°F. Line a large baking sheet with parchment paper.

In a large bowl, toss tomatoes with olive oil, honey, thyme, salt, and pepper or kelp. Arrange tomatoes on the sheet, cut side up, and bake about 60 to 75 minutes, until they shrivel and brown. Cool.

Preheat broiler. Place baguette slices on baking sheet. Broil for 30 seconds on each side.

Top bread with tomatoes. Drizzle with buckwheat honey, and sprinkle with basil.

··· **VARIATIONS** ···

▶ Use small vine-ripened tomatoes, cut into quarters, in place of grape or cherry tomatoes.

▶ Top with chopped green onions before eating.

> NOTE: Both clover and buckwheat are single varietal honeys, with distinctive color and taste. Each is made from the nectar of a single species of flower grown in a single place. To benefit from all of the nutrients and enzymes, look for raw honeys that haven't been processed or filtered. Buy local honey, which is healthiest of all. Go to www.honey locator.com to find someone in your area.

Sweet Potato–Chive Biscuits

YIELD: 10 to 12 servings
PREPARATION TIME: 30 minutes

Vitamins A and C, plus fiber and buttermilk's good bacteria in every crunchy bite.

1½ cups unbleached white flour
½ cup whole wheat flour
1 teaspoon baking powder
1 teaspoon salt
¼ cup unsalted butter or vegetarian margarine, room temperature

½ cup chopped chives
½ cup sweet potato, cooked and mashed
¾ cup buttermilk or kefir

Preheat oven to 450°F. Line a large baking sheet with parchment paper or lightly grease the pan.

Combine white and whole wheat flours, baking powder, and salt in a medium-size mixing bowl. Mix well. Cut butter or margarine into pea-size pieces, and combine with the flour mix. Use your fingers to work butter into flour mix until it has a coarse meal texture. Add chives.

Combine sweet potato and buttermilk (or kefir) in a small bowl, using a fork to combine. Combine this mixture with flour mixture, and stir until it forms a ball. Turn dough out onto a lightly floured surface, and knead for a minute. Pat dough to ½-inch thickness, and cut out rounds with a biscuit cutter or the mouth of a drinking glass. Combine scraps, pat down, roll out again, and cut into rounds.

Place rounds on prepared baking sheet, and bake 8 to 10 minutes until bottoms are golden brown.

VARIATIONS

▶ Add 2 tablespoons crushed flaxseeds.
▶ Add ¼ cup millet meal for added crunch.
▶ Substitute parsley, cilantro, or dill for chives.
▶ Cut into triangles or sticks instead of rounds.

Small Potato Chapatis

YIELD: 18 chapatis
PREPARATION TIME: 75 minutes

The basic flat bread of Northern India, used as a "spoon" to scoop up beans, vegetables, yogurt, and more, is best eaten hot off the griddle. This recipe is nutritionally enhanced with potato flour and sea vegetables.

1 cup whole wheat flour
½ cup potato flour
1 teaspoon kelp or dulse powder
  (optional)

1 teaspoon salt
¾ cup water
Oil for brushing

Combine both flours, kelp, and salt in a bowl. Stir in water until dough binds without sticking.

Grease a bowl, and turn the dough in it twice. Cover with a damp dish towel, and let rest for 1 hour. Knead again. Form dough into ½-inch-diameter balls. Flatten and roll into disks about ⅛ inch thick. Keep turning dough as you roll the disks out (using a lightly greased rolling pin). Cook the disks quickly on a very hot ungreased skillet until lightly browned on each side. Remove from heat, and cover with a damp cloth on each side to make chapatis puff up. Brush them with oil, and re-cover with a damp cloth until ready to serve.

··· **VARIATIONS** ···

▶ Use chickpea flour in place of the potato flour.
▶ Add 1 teaspoon dried rosemary or thyme before kneading.

Four-Grain Scones

YIELD: 16 scones

PREPARATION TIME: 30 minutes

*Make ahead, refrigerate, and then bake and serve
for hot-out-of-the-oven A.M. scones.*

¾ cup currants

1 cup unbleached all-purpose flour

½ cup whole wheat flour

½ cup soy grits or soy meal

½ cup rolled oats

1 teaspoon baking powder

1 tablespoon sugar

¼ teaspoon salt

6 tablespoons chilled unsalted
   butter or vegetarian margarine,
   cut into pieces

½ cup soy milk or low-fat dairy milk

¼ cup maple syrup

1 tablespoon soy lecithin granules

Preheat oven to 425°F. Grease baking sheet with oil. Place currants in a bowl, and cover them with boiling water.

Whisk together flours, meal, oats, baking powder, sugar, and salt in a large bowl. Add butter, and rub it into the flour mixture until it resembles coarse meal. Whisk together milk and maple syrup. Stir into flour mixture until dough is formed. Drain currants and add to dough.

Turn dough onto a well-floured cutting board, and knead until smooth. Pat or roll into a 1-inch-thick square. Sprinkle with soy lecithin granules. Cut into 16 scones using a 2-inch round cookie cutter or the mouth of a drinking glass. Place scones on baking sheet, and bake approximately 15 minutes, or until light brown.

··· **VARIATIONS** ···

▶ Use golden raisins, diced figs, or diced dates in place of currants.

▶ Use honey in place of maple syrup.

▶ Add ½ cup finely chopped raw nuts or seeds for crunch and added protein.

Portobello–Wild Rice Pancakes

YIELD: 4 servings

PREPARATION TIME: 20 minutes

*Rich in cancer-fighting selenium, portobellos have only
25 calories per cupful! Here they are paired with wild
rice, rich in vitamin B complex and protein.*

1 tablespoon olive oil

10 medium-size portobello mushrooms, washed and patted dry

1 teaspoon salt, divided

1 teaspoon minced fresh garlic

2 teaspoons lemon juice

4 eggs

⅓ cup unbleached flour

4 green onions, minced

1 cup cooked wild rice

¼ cup crumbled firm tofu or crumbled smoked tofu

Pinch black pepper or kelp or dulse powder

Heat large skillet over medium heat about 1 minute. Add olive oil and mushrooms, and stir-fry for 3 minutes. Add ½ teaspoon salt, and cook 3 minutes longer. Add garlic and lemon juice, and remove pan from heat.

Beat eggs in a separate bowl. Whisk in flour and remaining salt. Stir in cooked mushrooms. Add green onions, wild rice, tofu, pepper (or kelp or dulse), and combine well.

Wipe out skillet, grease it well again, and return to medium heat. When pan is hot, use a ½-cup measure to scoop batter into pan. Cook 2 to 3 minutes on each side, or until pancakes are golden brown. Remove to a warm platter. Serve with plain yogurt whipped with a bit of miso or spoon on Miso Vinaigrette (see page 148).

··· **VARIATIONS** ···

► Use shiitakes or button mushrooms in place of portobellos.

► Use crumbled feta cheese in place of tofu.

► Use kasha (buckwheat) in place of wild rice.

► For milder flavor, omit garlic, onions, or both.

Breakfast Berry Pops

YIELD: 8 servings

PREPARATION TIME: 10 minutes, plus 4 hours freezing time

This dessertlike A.M. meal rich in disease-fighting anthocyanins doubles as a dessert.

1½ cups fresh or thawed frozen strawberries

1 cup fresh or thawed frozen blueberries

1 cup fresh or thawed frozen raspberries

½ to 1 cup frozen white grape juice concentrate

½ cup plain yogurt or plain kefir

Puree ingredients in blender until smooth. Optional: strain through a fine sieve to remove seeds. Ladle mixture into ice pop molds or small paper cups, and freeze for 4 hours. If using cups, insert small plastic spoons or sticks after 30 minutes in freezer.

VARIATIONS

► Stir in ½ cup crushed walnuts or whole-grain cereal.

► Use 1 cup fresh or thawed frozen peach slices in place of 1 cup berries.

► Use two fruits instead of three.

Breakfast Pick-Up Sticks

YIELD: 4 servings

PREPARATION TIME: 45 minutes

Cranberries and blueberries are botanical cousins and partners in preventing dental plaque, cancer, and urinary tract infections.

7 cups whole-grain puffed cereal
¾ cup dried cranberries
¾ cup dried blueberries or raisins
1 teaspoon ground cinnamon

¾ cup brown rice syrup or honey
¾ cup almond butter
2 tablespoons soy margarine or
   unsalted butter

Stir together cereal, dried fruits, and cinnamon in large bowl.

Place syrup (or honey), almond butter, and margarine or butter in a microwave-safe measuring cup. Heat until contents have melted. Stir, and pour over cereal mixture. Stir to coat.

Wet your hands, and press mixture into 9-inch square baking pan. Freeze 30 minutes. Cut into 15 bars, and refrigerate.

··· VARIATIONS ···

▶ Add ½ cup raw nuts in place of dried fruit.
▶ Use pumpkin pie spice in place of cinnamon.
▶ Use peanut butter or cashew butter instead of almond butter.

SNACKS/SAUCES

Pepita Squash Spread

YIELD: 1½ cups

PREPARATION TIME: 25 minutes

Seven super immunity foods in one appetizer!

1½ cups cubed peeled butternut squash (about 1 pound)

1 teaspoon olive oil

½ cup diced onion

1½ teaspoons chopped fresh sage

¼ teaspoon salt

Pinch fresh ground pepper

2 garlic cloves, minced

Dash crushed red pepper

¼ cup chopped sun-dried tomatoes

2 tablespoons unsalted pumpkin seeds, toasted

Place squash in a medium saucepan; cover with water 2 inches above squash and bring to a boil. Cover, reduce heat, and cook 15 minutes or until tender. Drain.

Heat olive oil in a large skillet over medium-high heat. Add onion, and sauté until tender. Add sage and next four ingredients. Sauté 2 minutes longer. Cool.

Place squash, onion mix, and sun-dried tomatoes in food processor or blender, and process until smooth. Sprinkle with pumpkin seeds.

··· **VARIATIONS** ···

▶ Substitute another type of winter squash for the butternut.

▶ Use marjoram or basil in place of sage.

▶ Use flaxseeds or sunflower seeds in place of pumpkin seeds.

▶ Add kelp or dulse flakes or powder and/or 1 to 2 teaspoons soy lecithin granules.

Moroccan "Caviar"

YIELD: 1¼ cups

PREPARATION TIME: 15 minutes

No fish and no saturated fat, but plenty of healing seeds, herbs, and oil.

1 cup pitted Moroccan oil-cured olives

½ cup extra-virgin olive oil (more, if needed)

1 tablespoon ground cumin

2 teaspoons ground coriander

1 teaspoon cayenne pepper

2 cloves garlic, crushed

Place all ingredients in blender or food processor. Puree mixture, scraping down the sides. Add more oil if needed to produce a wet caviarlike paste.

Use immediately, or store well covered with a thin layer of oil in refrigerator for up to ten days.

··· **VARIATIONS** ···

▶ Use another type of olive in place of the Moroccan olives.

▶ Use oregano in place of coriander.

▶ Use sesame oil in place of olive oil.

Black-and-Brown
Health Hummus

YIELD: 8 servings

PREPARATION TIME: 75 minutes

Sweet potato gives this hummus its creamy richness and antioxidants. Serve it with broccoli florets, baby carrots, pepper strips, and other raw vegetables for dipping. Also, spread it on a whole-grain tortilla, top with sprouts, and roll up for a healthful wrap.

1 small sweet potato (about 5 or 6 ounces)

1 15-ounce can garbanzo beans (drained and rinsed)

2 tablespoons extra-virgin olive oil

½ cup chopped kalamata olives

2 medium cloves garlic, chopped

¼ teaspoon crushed red pepper flakes

⅓ cup fresh basil leaves, plus more for garnish

Salt and pepper, to taste

Minced sun-dried tomatoes for garnish

Wrap sweet potato in foil and bake at 400°F for about 1 hour, or until soft. Remove sweet potato from oven, unwrap, and let cool. Scoop out insides of sweet potato, and place in a food processor. Add garbanzos, olive oil, olives, garlic, and red pepper flakes. Puree until smooth. Add ⅓ cup of basil leaves, and pulse for 10 seconds.

Season with salt and pepper, and transfer to a serving bowl. Garnish with sun-dried tomatoes and whole basil leaves.

··· **VARIATIONS** ···

► Substitute another type of olive.

► Use hemp or sesame oil in place of olive oil.

► Use yam instead of sweet potato.

Cumin-Spiced Popcorn

YIELD: 6 servings
PREPARATION TIME: 15 minutes

Here's a healthy low-salt, low-fat munch.

¾ cup popcorn kernels
1 tablespoon olive oil
1 teaspoon ground coriander

1½ teaspoons ground cumin
1 teaspoon salt
¼ teaspoon ground red pepper

Combine all ingredients in a large, heavy pan. Cover and place over medium-high heat. When corn starts to pop, shake vigorously until all kernels are popped.

Eat while hot.

VARIATIONS

► Use grapeseed or canola oil in place of olive oil.
► Omit coriander, and sprinkle finished popcorn with minced cilantro.
► Use kelp or dulse powder in place of salt.
► Stir in ½ cup raw nuts to add omega-3 fats and protein.

Edamole

YIELD: 6 servings

PREPARATION TIME: 15 minutes

Use this edamame-based dip for vegetables and chips and as a spread for crackers.

¾ cup frozen shelled edamame, thawed

2 tablespoons olive oil

1 tablespoon fresh-squeezed lemon juice

3 tablespoons water

¾ teaspoon coarse salt

¼ teaspoon hot pepper sauce

1 garlic clove, halved

Combine ingredients in food processor or blender, and puree until smooth. Cover and chill.

··· **VARIATIONS** ···

▶ Add 1 tablespoon soy lecithin granules for more essential fatty acids.

▶ Increase garlic to 2 cloves for more bite.

▶ Use 1 tablespoon jalapeño pepper, diced, in place of hot sauce.

▶ Fold in 2 tablespoons plain yogurt.

Bluegrass Chips

YIELD: 18 pieces

PREPARATION TIME: 30 minutes

*Blue-green nori, the seaweed used to wrap sushi, also
makes a mineral-rich potato chip substitute.*

¼ cup brown rice syrup
3 tablespoons sesame oil
1 tablespoon dark sesame oil

¼ teaspoon cayenne pepper
3 sheets nori

Preheat oven to 350°F. Line two baking sheets with foil or parchment
paper.

Combine rice syrup and both sesame oils in a small bowl, and whisk to
blend. Stir in cayenne.

Tear each nori sheet into three strips, and place strips on baking
sheets. Coat each strip with the syrup-sesame mixture. Bake 10 minutes,
and remove from oven. Let stand 10 minutes to cool and crisp. Turn strips
over, brush again, and bake 10 more minutes. Let stand to crisp. Break
each strip in two.

Serve as a snack or with salads and soups.

Capsaicin Salsa

YIELD: 1 cup

PREPARATION TIME: 30 to 45 minutes

This salsa has vitamin C, beta-carotene, and plenty of no-fat zip.

4 large bell peppers, yellow, orange, or red

2 teaspoons cumin seeds or 2 teaspoons ground cumin

1-inch piece peeled fresh gingerroot

Salt and pepper, to taste

Grill or broil peppers, placing 4 inches from heat source and turning often until peppers blacken and collapse. Wrap in foil, and let cool.

If using whole cumin seeds, toast them in a dry skillet over medium heat, shaking pan. Remove from heat when seeds are fragrant. Grind seeds in a mill.

Remove core, skin, and seeds from cooled peppers. Place in food processor with cumin and gingerroot. Add salt, and puree. Taste, and adjust seasoning if needed.

Use as a dip for raw vegetables or breadsticks, serve as a sauce for a grilled entrée, or stir into hot rice. Salsa keeps in the refrigerator for several days or for one month in the freezer.

VARIATIONS

▶ Add raw or roasted garlic.

▶ Add ½ teaspoon fennel seed.

▶ Add ½ teaspoon kelp powder.

▶ Add ¼ cup chopped green or black olives.

Soy Sour Cream, Three Ways

YIELD: about 1 cup

PREPARATION TIME: 15 minutes, plus chilling time

Sour cream without the calories and cholesterol.

8 ounces soft tofu, drained

1½ tablespoons lemon juice

1 tablespoon olive or sunflower oil

¼ teaspoon salt

1 teaspoon soy lecithin granules

Pinch red pepper

Combine all ingredients, place in food processor or blender, and blend until smooth. Transfer to a refrigerator container with a tight lid, and chill before using. This keeps three to four days.

THREE WAYS

1. **Parsley Plus:** Add ¼ cup finely minced fresh parsley or cilantro before blending.
2. **Sea Veggie Punch:** Add ¼ cup roasted and crumbled sea vegetables, such as nori or dulse.
3. **Pepper Up:** Stir in ¼ cup diced red or yellow bell pepper before chilling.

Mustard Greens Pesto

YIELD: 4 to 6 servings

PREPARATION TIME: 15 minutes

Pesto with a plus: according to traditional Chinese medicine, greens cleanse and restore liver function; garlic boosts levels of detoxifying enzymes.

6 cloves garlic

1 cup walnuts

2 cups (packed) fresh mustard
    greens, washed and dried

½ teaspoon kosher sea salt

3 tablespoons extra-virgin olive oil

Place garlic in a food processor and mince. Add walnuts, and process until finely ground. Add mustard greens and salt, and process until a thick paste forms. Slowly drizzle in olive oil, and process until smooth.

  Swirl this tasty pesto into broth, spread on crusty whole-grain bread, or mix into whole wheat noodles or rice.

··· VARIATIONS ··

► Use cashews in place of walnuts, or combine ½ cup almonds and ½ cup unsalted peanuts instead of walnuts.

► Use sesame oil in place of olive oil.

► Add ½ teaspoon kelp powder for more trace minerals.

► Add a few drops hot pepper sauce for more bite.

Olive-Oil Mayonnaise

YIELD: 1 cup
PREPARATION TIME: 10 minutes

Make your own better-than butter spread in just minutes.

....   —   ....

1 large organic egg yolk
1 teaspoon Dijon mustard or dry
   mustard
1 cup olive oil, divided

Salt to taste
Pinch cayenne pepper
1 to 2 tablespoons fresh-squeezed
   lemon juice or vinegar

In a mixing bowl (if you're mixing by hand), the bowl of an electric mixer, a blender, or a food processor, place the egg yolk, mustard, and a couple of tablespoons of oil and whisk or beat until pale yellow. Add the remaining oil: a few drops at a time at first, while whisking or with the machine running, and then in a steady, thin stream. Once the mixture starts to thicken, you may add the oil slightly faster, until all of it is incorporated. Scrape down the sides of the bowl; add the salt, cayenne, and lemon juice (or vinegar), and beat in briefly. Taste and adjust seasoning. If mayonnaise is too thick, beat in a tablespoon or so of hot tap water.

> NOTE: If the mixture separates or curdles, get a new bowl and another egg yolk and beat in the old mixture. Or pour all but 1 tablespoon out of the bowl you're using. Add 1 tablespoon of water to the tablespoon of failed mixture, and whisk or beat. Continue to whisk or beat while adding the rest of the separated mayonnaise gradually.

   Transfer to a clean container, seal, and store in refrigerator. Use up within five days.

⋯ VARIATIONS ⋯

▶ Experiment with different flavors of olive oil and vinegar.
▶ Add in chopped fresh herbs (e.g., thyme, basil, parsley, or dill).

Pecan-Mint Pesto

YIELD: 1 cup

PREPARATION TIME: 10 minutes

Get your pecan intake up and your cholesterol down with this fragrant dip or bread spread (or thin for sauce).

¼ cup pecans

4 tablespoons chopped fresh mint

Juice of ½ lemon

3 garlic cloves, chopped

Pinch sea salt

2 tablespoons extra-virgin olive oil

In a food processor, finely chop pecans. Add mint, lemon juice, garlic, and salt, and process until well blended. With processor still running, slowly add oil and process until smooth.

··· VARIATIONS ··

▶ Use cashews in place of pecans.

▶ Substitute basil for the mint.

▶ Add 1 teaspoon kelp or dulse powder.

Hot Peanut Dip-and-Dribble Sauce

YIELD: 1 cup

PREPARATION TIME: 15 minutes

Give your rice or rutabaga more bite and more
B vitamins with this two-way sauce.

½ cup smooth natural peanut butter
1 tablespoon minced garlic
¼ cup tamari or low-sodium soy sauce
¼ cup water (or as needed)
1 tablespoon rice vinegar

1 teaspoon Asian chili paste
1 teaspoon sugar or natural sweetener such as honey
2 tablespoons finely chopped cilantro

In a small bowl, combine everything but the cilantro. Blend until smooth. Taste and adjust seasonings (add more liquid if needed).

Stir in cilantro before using. Use as a dipping sauce or as a dressing for vegetables or grains. Keeps up to five days.

VARIATIONS

▶ Use almond butter in place of peanut butter.
▶ Add 1 teaspoon lemon juice, ½ teaspoon lemon zest, or both.
▶ For a crunchy dip, use crunchy-style peanut butter.
▶ Add 1 teaspoon grated onions or chopped green onions.

Fig Vinaigrette

YIELD: about ⅓ cup

PREPARATION TIME: 15 minutes

Give your greens a fruity, garlicky finish that benefits four immune centers.

½ cup balsamic vinegar

5 dried Black Mission figs, stemmed and coarsely chopped

6 tablespoons water

1 tablespoon fresh-squeezed lemon juice

2 tablespoons minced shallots

1 teaspoon minced fresh thyme

1 garlic clove, minced

1 tablespoon extra-virgin olive oil

Pinch salt

Combine balsamic vinegar and figs in small saucepan over high heat, and bring to a boil. Reduce heat and simmer until reduced to ⅓ cup.

Combine fig mixture, water, and lemon juice in blender, and process until smooth. Place fig mixture in small bowl. Stir in shallots, thyme, garlic, olive oil, and salt. Stir well, using a whisk.

Spoon over tossed greens or grains.

Citrusy Carrot-Ginger Dressing

YIELD: 1 cup

PREPARATION TIME: 10 minutes

Here are five super immunity ingredients in one simple raw salad sauce.

½ cup fresh or canned carrot juice

2 teaspoons orange juice, fresh-squeezed or bottled

2 teaspoons lemon juice, fresh-squeezed or bottled

4 tablespoons sesame oil

3 tablespoons light-colored miso paste

1 tablespoon peeled and grated fresh gingerroot

1 teaspoon honey

½ teaspoon lemon zest

½ teaspoon orange zest

½ teaspoon low-sodium soy sauce

Dash pepper or kelp powder

In a blender or food processor, combine everything and blend until smooth.

Use on any tossed greens, on shredded cabbage, or over cold, cooked whole grains.

··· **VARIATIONS** ···

▶ Use walnut oil or avocado oil in place of sesame oil, or substitute flaxseed oil.

▶ Add 2 tablespoons toasted sesame seeds or toasted sunflower seeds.

▶ Stir in ¼ cup sprouted lentils or sprouted peas.

Miso Vinaigrette

YIELD: 1 cup

PREPARATION TIME: 15 minutes

Dress your greens with miso for more bone-building protein, vitamin K, and manganese.

2 tablespoons miso paste, red or brown

2 tablespoons whole-grain mustard

½ cup low-sodium vegetable stock

2 tablespoons fresh-squeezed lemon juice

2 tablespoons fresh-squeezed lime juice

½ cup extra-virgin olive oil

2 teaspoons peeled and minced fresh gingerroot

1 scallion, minced

1 teaspoon chopped chives

3 sprigs parsley, chopped

In a mixing bowl, mix together miso and mustard. Whisk in the vegetable stock, lemon juice, and lime juice. Add the oil in a slow, steady stream while whisking vigorously until dressing is emulsified. With a spatula, stir in gingerroot, scallion, chives, and parsley.

Dribble over mixed greens, steamed vegetables, or cooked pasta.

VARIATIONS

▶ Use fresh cilantro in place of parsley.

▶ Add soy lecithin granules while whisking and adding oil.

▶ Sprinkle with sesame seeds before serving.

Pink Dressing for Greens

YIELD: 1 cup

PREPARATION TIME: 10 minutes

*Savor as a vegetable or chip dip or sandwich spread;
to use as a soup, dilute further and chill.*

1 red bell pepper, cut in chunks
½ lemon, seeded, peeled, and
   chopped
1 teaspoon low-sodium soy sauce,
   tamari, or liquid aminos (a
   soybean-based all-purpose
   seasoning)

1 cup grated beets
½ cup tahini
1 teaspoon paprika

In a blender, combine red pepper, lemon, and soy sauce (or tamari or aminos), and blend until smooth. Add beets, and blend again. Add tahini, paprika, and enough water for the desired consistency.

VARIATIONS

▶ Add 1 firm tomato and a pinch of cayenne pepper.
▶ Add ¼ cup chopped fresh parsley or cilantro.
▶ Add 1 tablespoon yogurt along with the tahini.

SALADS

Spinach-Apple Salad with Maple Dressing

YIELD: 6 servings

PREPARATION TIME: 15 minutes

Try this sweet and sour, fruit and vegetable toss-up.

1 tablespoon maple syrup
1 teaspoon red wine vinegar
¼ teaspoon Dijon mustard
1 tablespoon extra-virgin olive oil
1 tablespoon chopped fresh chives
Pinch salt and pepper

2½ cups julienned Granny Smith apple
¼ cup sliced red onion
6 ounces (about) baby spinach leaves

Combine first three ingredients in a small bowl; stir well with a whisk and gradually add oil. Add chives, salt, and pepper, and blend.

Combine apple, onion, and spinach in a large bowl. Drizzle with vinaigrette, and toss to serve.

VARIATIONS

► Fold in ½ cup sliced mushrooms.
► Use parsley or cilantro in place of chives.
► Use Golden Delicious apples in place of Granny Smiths.
► To serve as a whole-meal salad, add 1 cup of black beans or diced tofu.

Watermelon and Tomato Salad

YIELD: 4 servings

PREPARATION TIME: 20 minutes

A first course rich in anticancer lycopene.

2½ cups seedless watermelon cut in 1-inch cubes

1½ cups sliced cherry tomatoes

½ cup finely crumbled blue cheese, feta, or nondairy equivalent

½ cup minced green onions

Salt or kelp or dulse powder, to taste

2 tablespoons extra-virgin olive oil

2 tablespoons balsamic or rice wine vinegar

Pinch ground red pepper

½ cup finely minced parsley or cilantro

Combine watermelon, tomato, cheese, green onions, and salt (or kelp or dulse) in bowl. Blend together oil, vinegar, and red pepper. Combine two mixtures, and top with cilantro or parsley.

VARIATIONS

▶ Use a combination of red and yellow watermelon.

▶ Add toasted flaxseeds or pumpkin seeds to dressing.

▶ Add ½ cup avocado slices before serving.

Bitter Greens Salad

YIELD: 6 servings

PREPARATION TIME: 15 minutes

To prepare this salad ahead, whisk together the dressing ingredients, and then refrigerate. Combine the greens, and refrigerate separately; toss with the dressing and garnish with cheese right before serving.

DRESSING

1 tablespoon cider vinegar

1½ teaspoons chopped fresh thyme

1½ teaspoons extra-virgin olive oil

1 teaspoon Dijon mustard

¼ teaspoon salt or kelp powder

¼ teaspoon freshly ground black pepper

½ cup chopped onion, yellow or red

REMAINING SALAD INGREDIENTS

4 cups torn mustard greens

2 cups torn radicchio

1 cup torn Belgian endive

¼ cup (1 ounce) shaved Parmigiano-Reggiano cheese for garnish

To prepare dressing, combine first seven ingredients in a large bowl, stirring with a whisk. Add radicchio and endive; toss to coat.

Arrange on a platter, and top with cheese.

··· **VARIATIONS** ···

▶ Use dandelion greens in place of mustard greens.

▶ Use red cabbage (shredded) instead of radicchio.

▶ Use balsamic or rice wine vinegar in place of cider vinegar.

▶ Use ½ cup broccoli sprouts instead of cheese topping.

Marinated Kale Salad

YIELD: 6 servings

PREPARATION TIME: 15 minutes

*Trade empty-calorie iceberg for Vitamin A-, C-, and
K-rich kale. Only this variety is safe to eat raw; check
with your nearest health food store for availability.*

2 tablespoons fresh-squeezed
   lemon juice
4 tablespoons extra-virgin olive oil
   or flax oil
2 teaspoons minced garlic
1 teaspoon sea salt

1 bunch Tuscan kale (also known
   as black or lacinato kale), stems
   removed, washed and dried
   thoroughly, and sliced crossways
   into 1-inch strips

In a mixing bowl, combine lemon juice, olive oil, garlic, and salt; whisk to
blend. Add kale, and toss until leaves are coated. Serve immediately or
store, covered and refrigerated, for up to one day.

VARIATIONS

► Toss in 1 cup lentil or bean sprouts.
► Add red onion slices.
► Fold in ¼ cup toasted nori (sea vegetables).
► Sprinkle with soy lecithin granules, hemp seeds, or sesame seeds.

Raw Slaw 1 (with Chard)

YIELD: 6 servings

PREPARATION TIME: 30 minutes

Tender Swiss chard leaves are ideal in raw cuisine recipes because they are not only milder than other leafy greens like kale and collards but also less prone to tearing and wilting than spinach.

13 Swiss chard leaves, stems removed, sliced into ¼-inch-thick ribbons

1 large Asian pear, peeled and grated (3 cups)

4 large navel oranges, peeled, segmented, and chopped (3 cups)

3 large carrots, grated (2 cups)

⅓ cup chopped cilantro

⅔ cup raw cashews

¼ cup fresh-squeezed orange juice

2 teaspoons sesame oil

¼ cup rice wine vinegar

Pinch powdered red pepper

1 teaspoon peeled and minced fresh gingerroot

Toss together chard, Asian pear, oranges, carrots, and cilantro in bowl. Set aside.

Blend cashews, orange juice, and sesame oil in blender 15 seconds, or until nuts are finely ground. Add rice wine vinegar, red pepper, and gingerroot, and blend 10 seconds more or until smooth and frothy. Add to chard mixture, and toss to coat.

Raw Slaw 2 (with Kale)

YIELD: 4 servings

PREPARATION TIME: 20 minutes

*All kale is not created equal, and only this variety is edible raw.
Check with your nearest health food store for this variety.*

1 thin slice country bread (whole wheat or rye, for instance)
½ garlic clove, finely chopped
¼ cup finely grated hard cheese, more for garnish
3 tablespoons extra-virgin olive oil, more for garnish
1 tablespoon fresh-squeezed lemon juice
¼ teaspoon salt
⅛ teaspoon red pepper flakes
Freshly ground black pepper to taste
1 bunch Tuscan kale (also known as black or lacinato kale), bottom 2 inches trimmed and sliced into ¾-inch strips (4 or 5 cups)

Toast bread until golden on both sides. Tear into small pieces, and grind in food processor until mixture becomes coarse crumbs.

Using a garlic press or with back of a knife, turn garlic into a paste. Transfer garlic to a small bowl. Add ¼ cup cheese, 3 tablespoons oil, lemon juice, salt, red pepper flakes, and black pepper; whisk to combine. Pour dressing over kale, and toss well to thoroughly combine. The dressing will be thick and require lots of tossing to properly coat leaves.

Let salad sit for 5 minutes. Serve topped with bread crumbs, additional cheese, and a drizzle of oil.

VARIATIONS

▶ Toss in a heaping handful of soybean or mung bean sprouts for antioxidants and isoflavones.
▶ Use red chard in place of kale.
▶ Fold in slices of firm spicy tofu or ½ cup of cooked black beans.
▶ Add ½ cup halved green or black olives.

Immunity Toss-Up 1

YIELD: 2 servings

PREPARATION TIME: 20 minutes

Did you know that grapefruit juice contains more nutrients per calorie than any other fruit juice? Fill up on seed, vegetable, and fruit phytonutrients with this midday or p.m. salad.

2 pink grapefruits

2 tablespoons olive oil

1 tablespoon minced shallots

1 teaspoon low-sodium soy sauce or tamari

½ teaspoon honey

¼ teaspoon sesame oil

1 teaspoon grated, peeled fresh gingerroot

1 teaspoon coriander seeds, cracked

Salt and pepper or kelp or dulse powder to taste

2 cups of mixed baby greens

1 small avocado, pitted, peeled, and halved

Peel the first grapefruit, and slice crosswise into four slices. Cut second grapefruit in half, and juice. Set aside 3 tablespoons.

Whisk juice and olive oil together with remaining ingredients except for greens and avocado. Taste and adjust seasoning with salt and pepper or kelp or dulse powder. Toss greens with 2 tablespoons dressing and divide into two servings.

Place grapefruit slices and avocado alongside greens, and spoon on remaining dressing.

VARIATIONS

► Use white grapefruit or pomelo in place of pink.
► Replace shallots with green onions.
► Use toasted pine nuts in place of coriander.
► Use baby spinach in place of greens.
► Use kiwi slices in place of avocado.

Immunity Toss-Up 2

YIELD: 4 to 6 servings

PREPARATION TIME: 15 minutes

Pomegranate seeds are crunchy, cardio-protective, and rich in vitamin C.

2 cups very thinly sliced fennel bulb or celery root

3 tablespoons extra-virgin olive oil, divided

¼ teaspoon coarse salt, divided

6 cups arugula

½ cup thinly sliced green onions

¼ cup slivered mint leaves

1 tablespoon balsamic vinegar

½ cup pomegranate seeds

Black pepper to taste

Toss fennel or celery root with 1 tablespoon olive oil in a medium bowl, and sprinkle with half the salt.

Combine arugula, green onions, mint, vinegar, and 2 tablespoons olive oil in a large bowl. Season with remaining salt and pepper as needed.

Divide greens on salad plates. Top with fennel or celery root and sprinkle with pomegranate seeds.

··· **VARIATIONS** ···

▶ Substitute jicama for fennel.

▶ Use crumbled toasted sea vegetables for salt.

▶ Substitute crushed goji berries or currants for pomegranate seeds.

Power Kraut

YIELD: 4 servings

PREPARATION TIME: 15 minutes

Balsamic vinegar replaces the kraut-fermenting process in this six-vegetable slaw.

2 cups of shredded red cabbage or radicchio

1 cup shredded green cabbage or bok choy

1 large carrot, grated or shredded

1 red bell pepper, sliced

2 green onions, sliced

½ bunch fresh parsley, chopped

¼ cup balsamic vinegar

3 tablespoons water

1 tablespoon flaxseed oil or extra-virgin olive oil

½ teaspoon red pepper flakes

1 teaspoon caraway seeds

½ teaspoon low-sodium soy sauce, tamari, or liquid aminos such as Bragg's

Combine all the vegetables, and toss with the remaining ingredients. Allow flavors to mingle and develop for at least one hour.

Serve cold or at room temperature.

··· **VARIATIONS** ···

▶ Substitute slivers of seeded tomato for the red bell pepper.

▶ Add slivered or shredded turnip or fennel bulb.

▶ Substitute shredded or chopped celery for carrot.

Spicy Granny Smith Salad

YIELD: 4 servings

PREPARATION TIME: 30 minutes

Juicy, spicy, and crunchy, here are six super immunity foods in one dish.

6 Granny Smith apples, peeled and grated

¼ cup plus 2 tablespoons fresh-squeezed lime juice

1 bunch green onions, chopped

2 cloves garlic, minced

2 teaspoons low-sodium soy sauce or tamari

1 teaspoon chili paste (such as the Asian sambal oelek)

1 cup halved cherry tomatoes

I small bunch watercress

Toss grated apples with ¼ cup lime juice to prevent oxidation; add green onions.

Stir together remaining lime juice, garlic, soy sauce (or tamari), and chili paste. Add to grated apples, and toss well. Fold in cherry tomatoes.

Serve on a bed of watercress.

··· **VARIATIONS** ···

▶ Stir in ¼ cup chopped black olives with tomatoes.

▶ Stir in ½ cup cooked, cooled sea vegetables such as hijiki or arame.

▶ Add diced jicama or water chestnuts for added crunch.

Fruit and Root Spinach Salad

YIELD: 8 servings

PREPARATION TIME: 30 minutes

Empower your greens with anti-inflammatory grapefruit and ginger.

2 pink grapefruits
1 bag or bunch baby spinach
    leaves
¼ sliced almonds

DRESSING
3 tablespoons grapefruit juice

3 tablespoons sesame or extra-
    virgin olive oil
1 teaspoon tomato sauce
1 teaspoon peeled and minced fresh
    gingerroot
1 teaspoon spicy mustard
1 clove garlic, minced

Peel grapefruit, remove membrane, and break into segments. Combine grapefruit juice with oil, tomato sauce, gingerroot, mustard, and garlic. Combine spinach, nuts, and grapefruit segments in large salad bowl, and toss with dressing.

VARIATIONS

▶ Use Ugli fruit or a pomelo in place of grapefruit.
▶ Use mesclun instead of baby spinach.
▶ Substitute toasted sunflower seeds for the almonds.
▶ Sprinkle with soy lecithin granules and toasted nori.

SOUPS

Beta-Carotene Bisque

YIELD: 4 to 5 servings

PREPARATION TIME: 45 minutes

Carrots, leeks, and sweet potatoes are great solo but even greater together.

2 teaspoons olive oil

1 medium-size leek, white part only, cut in half lengthwise, rinsed well between the layers, and thinly sliced

1 medium carrot, chopped

1 pound sweet potatoes or yams, peeled and cubed

1-inch piece fresh gingerroot, peeled and finely chopped, plus 1 teaspoon peeled and grated fresh gingerroot for garnish

4 cups of vegetable broth, preferably homemade

Salt to taste

1 tablespoon chopped fresh cilantro for garnish

Heat the oil in a heavy 4-quart saucepan over medium-high heat. Add the leek and carrot, and cook, stirring, until they begin to soften (2 to 3 minutes). Stir in the sweet potatoes and chopped gingerroot. Add the broth, and bring to a boil. Cover the saucepan, reduce the heat to low, and simmer until the sweet potatoes are soft, about 30 minutes. Transfer the soup to a food processor or blender, or use an immersion blender, and process until smooth. Pour the soup back into the saucepan, adding ½ cup more broth or water if it seems too thick. Season with salt to taste.

Reheat before serving. Just before serving, stir in the grated ginger-root and garnish each serving with some of the cilantro.

··· VARIATIONS ·····

▶ Use butternut squash in place of sweet potato.

▶ Use parsley or dill in place of cilantro.

▶ Add 1 clove of garlic , chopped.

▶ Substitute 1 small yellow onion in place of leek.

Cream of Wheat Berry Soup

YIELD: 4 to 6 servings

PREPARATION TIME: 45 minutes

*High-protein, high-fiber wheat berries make this
soup one up on cream of mushroom.*

½ cup dried porcini mushrooms

Boiling water to cover

6 cups vegetable stock

1 tablespoon olive oil or canola oil

1 medium onion, chopped

2 medium carrots, chopped

1 stalk celery, chopped

2 to 3 garlic cloves (to taste), minced or put through a press

1 teaspoon fresh thyme leaves, or ½ teaspoon dried thyme (more to taste)

1½ cups wheat berries

Salt, preferably sea salt, to taste

Freshly ground black pepper, to taste

2 tablespoons dry sherry

3 tablespoons chopped fresh parsley

Place the dried mushrooms in a bowl, and pour boiling water to cover. Place a small plate or saucer on top to push the mushrooms under the water. Steep 30 minutes. Drain into a bowl through a strainer lined with cheesecloth, and rinse mushrooms thoroughly. Squeeze dry, and chop. Add mushroom-soaking liquid to stock.

Heat the oil in a large, heavy-bottomed soup pot over medium-low heat, and add the onion. Cook while stirring, until the onion begins to soften. Add the carrots and celery. Cook, stirring, about 5 minutes more. Stir in the garlic, thyme, and mushrooms. Stir together; then stir in the wheat berries. Add stock, salt, and pepper, and bring to a boil. Reduce heat, cover, and simmer 1 hour, until the wheat berries are tender.

Remove 2 cups of the soup, and puree in a blender or a food processor fitted with the steel blade. Stir the puree back into the soup, along with the sherry. Add salt to taste and lots of freshly ground black pepper. Heat through, taste, and adjust seasonings. Sprinkle on the parsley, and serve.

▶ Substitute rye berries or whole barley for wheat berries.

▶ Use salt-free salt or kelp powder in place of salt.

▶ Use white wine in place of sherry.

▶ Stir in 1 to 2 teaspoons green foods powder before blending.

▶ Top with sprouts.

Minted White Gazpacho

YIELD: 6 servings

PREPARATION TIME: 20 minutes, plus chilling time

Improve your complexion and your blood pressure with a soup rich in silica and fiber.

2 slices sandwich bread, crusts removed, soaked in cold water

4 large cucumbers (about 3 pounds), peeled and seeded, divided

⅓ cup fresh mint leaves, plus sprigs for garnish

2 tablespoons olive oil

2 tablespoons sherry vinegar

2 cloves garlic, chopped (about 2 teaspoons)

½ teaspoon hot pepper sauce

Salt to taste

2 tablespoons snipped fresh chives for garnish

Drain bread in colander, lightly press out excess water, and place in blender. Cut 3 cucumbers into ½-inch dice, and place in the blender along with mint, oil, vinegar, garlic, and hot pepper sauce. Process mixture until thick and smooth.

Cut remaining cucumber into ½-inch dice, and stir into soup; season with salt. Refrigerate 1 to 2 hours. Taste, and adjust seasonings as necessary.

Pour into chilled bowls, garnish with chives and mint sprigs, and serve.

··· **VARIATIONS** ···

▶ Use summer squash in place of cukes.

▶ Use basil in place of mint.

▶ Stir in cubed tofu or cubes of feta cheese to add protein.

▶ Top with alfalfa, clover, or radish sprouts.

Big Bowl Borscht

YIELD: 6 servings

PREPARATION TIME: 2 hours

Beef up the health of your heart and help cleanse your liver with beets.

....   ⌒   ....

4 medium-size red beets (greens removed and saved for another use), scrubbed

2 medium-size onions, cut in half and thinly sliced

2 cups shredded green cabbage

1 cup canned chopped tomatoes, with their juices

4 cups vegetable broth

Salt or sea salt to taste

Preheat oven to 450°F. Wrap the beets in two layers of aluminum foil. Place on the middle shelf in the oven, and roast for 1 hour. Remove from oven, and unwrap. When beets are cool enough to handle, use a sharp knife to peel and cut into 1-inch cubes. Set aside.

In a heavy 4-quart saucepan, combine the beets with onions, cabbage, tomatoes, and broth, and season with salt to taste. Reduce heat, partially cover saucepan and simmer for 1 hour.

Serve in preheated soup bowls. Top with sprouted lentils, clover, or alfalfa. Accompany with whole-grain crackers.

··· **VARIATIONS** ···

▶ Serve with tofu croutons.

▶ Serve with date-nut bread.

Zucchini-Pear
Summer-Winter Soup

YIELD: 4 servings

PREPARATION TIME: 25 minutes

Four vegetables pureed with a pear for an any-season nutrition booster.

3 tablespoons butter or extra-virgin olive oil, or a combination

1 medium carrot, peeled and diced

1 medium onion, diced

1 medium potato, preferably high starch (russet or baking), peeled and diced

½ teaspoon fresh thyme leaves, or a pinch of dried thyme

Salt and black pepper to taste

4 medium zucchini, trimmed and diced

2 medium ripe (but still firm) pears, peeled, cored, and diced

4 cups vegetable stock or water

Mint leaves for garnish (optional)

Put butter, oil, or combination in a large skillet over medium heat. When butter melts or oil is hot, cook carrot, onion, potato, and thyme with a healthy sprinkling of salt and pepper. Stir occasionally, adjusting the heat so vegetables don't brown. When onion is soft, add zucchini and cook 10 to 15 minutes. Add pear, and cook 5 minutes more. Add liquid and bring to a boil; taste and adjust seasoning.

Cool mixture; then puree. Serve cold, or reheat and serve hot. Garnish with mint.

VARIATIONS

► Use yellow summer squash or chayote in place of zucchini.

► Use leeks or shallots in place of onion.

► Garnish with pea sprouts or grated radish.

Sweet Potato Slurpy

YIELD: 4 servings

PREPARATION TIME: 45 minutes

This makes for a great soup now, sauce later.

1 tablespoon unsalted vegetarian margarine or omega-3 butter

I large stalk celery, chopped

I fresh sage leaf chopped

1 small yellow onion, chopped

1 parsnip, peeled and chopped

1 carrot, peeled and diced

4 clementines

3 medium sweet potatoes, peeled and chopped

2 tablespoons white wine

Pinch nutmeg

Pinch powdered ginger

2½ cups vegetable stock

2 tablespoons nondairy heavy cream

Heat butter in large pot over medium heat, and add celery, sage, onion, parsnip, and carrot, cooking until onion has softened, about 5 minutes.

Grate zest from clementines' peels; set aside. Cut clementines in half, and then squeeze to make juice; set aside.

Add sweet potatoes, and cook for 2 minutes; add juice from clementines, nutmeg, wine, and ginger. Add stock, reduce heat to low, and cook puree mixture.

Before serving as soup, add zest and cream to each bowl, or use as a dip for raw vegetables.

Protein Pea Soup

YIELD: 4 to 5 servings
PREPARATION TIME: 30 minutes

Did you know that peas have more protein than any other green vegetable? For even more protein, add tofu cubes, plain, smoked, or flavored, to this soup.

1 small leek, split lengthwise, thinly sliced

3 cups fresh or frozen and thawed peas

2 stalks celery, diced

1 teaspoon lemon zest

2 cups plain soy milk or skim dairy milk

2 cups spring water

2 tablespoons white wine

Salt and pepper or kelp powder, to taste

2 to 3 green onions, thinly sliced on the diagonal, for garnish

Lemon slices for garnish

Flaxseeds or hemp seeds for garnish

Place leek, peas, celery, and lemon zest in a soup pot. Add soy milk, water, wine, and pinch of salt. Cover, and bring to a boil over medium heat. Reduce heat to low, and cook for 15 minutes. Season to taste with salt and pepper (or kelp powder), and simmer for 5 minutes. Transfer soup by the ladleful to a food processor or blender, and puree until smooth. Return soup to the pot, and simmer 2 minutes longer.

Serve garnished with green onions, lemon, and flaxseeds or hemp seeds.

··· VARIATIONS ···

▶ Substitute asparagus for peas.

▶ Use lime in place of lemon.

▶ Use a mild low-sodium vegetable broth in place of water.

Lentil-Dulse Soup

YIELD: 4 to 5 servings

PREPARATION TIME: 45 minutes

Dulse and lentils for protein without meat.

2 onions, chopped fine

2 cloves of garlic, chopped fine

2 tablespoons grapeseed or olive oil

1 cup red lentils

5 cups low-sodium vegetable broth

1 ounce dried dulse, chopped

Salt and freshly ground black pepper
  to taste

Sauté onions and garlic in oil for 3 to 4 minutes. Rinse and add lentils and broth. Bring to a boil. Add dulse to saucepan. Turn heat to a low simmer; cover pan and simmer 20 to 30 minutes, stirring now and then. Add salt and pepper. Taste and adjust seasoning.

··· **VARIATIONS** ···

▶ Substitute green or black lentils for red.

▶ Use kelp powder in place of pepper.

▶ Increase dulse to 2 ounces.

▶ Add 1 cup of buckwheat noodles or cooked brown rice before serving.

SIDE DISHES

Mashed Potatoes Plus

YIELD: 4 to 5 servings

PREPARATION TIME: 45 minutes

Lower on the glycemic index than regular mashed potatoes and higher in potassium and folate.

3 pounds russet potatoes, peeled and quartered (3 to 4 medium potatoes)

1 pound parsnips, peeled and cut into 2-inch pieces

½ cup plain nonfat yogurt, at room temperature

2 tablespoons unsalted butter

1 tablespoon chopped chives or green onions for garnish

Salt and black pepper to taste

Cook potatoes and parsnips for about 30 minutes in a large pot of boiling salted water. Drain in a colander, and return to the pot. Mash the potatoes and parsnips, folding in yogurt and butter until mixture is smooth. Add salt and pepper. Garnish with chives or green onions.

··· **VARIATIONS** ··

▶ Stir in 1 tablespoon ground flaxseeds or soy lecithin granules.

▶ Add 1 teaspoon kelp or dulse powder in place of salt and pepper.

▶ Use soy half-and-half in place of yogurt, or use kefir.

Basil Couscous with Squash

YIELD: 4 servings

PREPARATION TIME: 45 minutes

You can prepare this year-round recipe in the summer with yellow summer squash and zucchini. Come autumn and winter, try buttercup squash. Try adding parsley for extra flavor.

¾ cup water

1 teaspoon extra-virgin olive oil

¾ teaspoon salt or kelp powder

1 cup basil leaves, cut in strips

½ cup quick-cooking couscous

2 cups zucchini or summer squash, cut in ¼-inch cubes, steamed until tender

In a medium saucepan, bring water to a boil. Stir in the olive oil, salt (or kelp powder), and basil. Boil until basil is wilted. Add couscous, and remove pan from burner. Let stand covered for about 5 minutes.

Fluff couscous with fork; then combine with steamed squash. Serve warm.

VARIATIONS

▶ Sprinkle with flaxseed.

▶ Add 1 tablespoon of soy lecithin granules or flakes to couscous.

▶ Substitute 2 cups steamed buttercup squash for a winter variation.

Toaster Oven Tomatoes

YIELD: 24 servings

A lycopene-rich snack that's not sugary or fattening.

PREPARATION TIME: 10 minutes, plus drying time

1 to 2 cups halved ripe (but not too   2 tablespoons olive oil
   ripe) cherry tomatoes

Brush cherry tomatoes with olive oil, and arrange on the baking sheet of the toaster oven. Set oven to 150°F. Let tomatoes dry for 8 hours or overnight. Place in plastic bags or pack in oil to keep longer.

To prepare in a conventional oven: brush tomatoes with olive oil, place on a baking sheet, and dry in a 150°F oven for 8 hours or longer.

VARIATIONS

▶ Try a combination of red and yellow cherry tomatoes or a combination of red, yellow, and green full-sized tomatoes.
▶ In dry climates, tomatoes may be dried outside on cookie sheets, covered with thin cheesecloth. Place where there is good circulation and a warm, not hot, sun. Turn every 8 hours until completely dry.

Peas Twice

YIELD: 6 servings

PREPARATION TIME: less than 10 minutes

*Protein, little fat, and plenty of vitamin K for
bones. Good as a side dish or snack.*

¾ pound sugar snap peas, trimmed

2 cups fresh or thawed frozen petite green peas

1½ tablespoons unsalted butter, softened

¼ teaspoon kosher or sea salt

2 tablespoons finely chopped fresh mint

Steam snap peas covered for 2 minutes. Add green peas, and steam for an additional 2 minutes. Combine peas, butter, and salt in a large bowl. Toss to coat. Sprinkle with mint.

··· **VARIATIONS** ···

▶ Serve over shredded crinkly cabbage or watercress.

▶ Fold in ½ cup of sprouted peas or lentils.

▶ Drizzle with extra-virgin olive oil.

Peanut Butter Broccoli

YIELD: 4 servings

PREPARATION TIME: 30 minutes

Serve this family-friendly dish at room temperature or chilled.

1 large bunch broccoli (about 1½ pounds), separated into florets, stems cut into spears

DIPPING SAUCE
¼ cup peanut butter
1 cup hot water
1 teaspoon fresh-squeezed or bottled lemon juice

Place a vegetable steamer in a deep pot filled with water, add broccoli, and cover. Bring water to a boil, reduce heat to medium, and cook for 3 to 5 minutes until broccoli is green and tender. Drain and rinse broccoli under cold water to cool. Pat dry.

For dipping sauce, whisk peanut butter with the hot water. Stir in lemon juice.

Pour dipping sauce in a small bowl, and arrange broccoli around sauce, or top the broccoli with the sauce and serve.

··· **VARIATIONS**

► Substitute almond, cashew, or sesame butter for peanut butter.
► Use broccoli raab in place of broccoli.
► Top sauce with toasted sesame seeds before serving.

Pink Roasted Beets

YIELD: 4 servings

PREPARATION TIME: 1 hour

Beets made better—with a citrus glaze.

3 pounds beets, greens trimmed

3 tablespoons water

1 cup fresh-squeezed pink grapefruit juice

2 tablespoons maple syrup

1 tablespoon rice vinegar

1 tablespoon cornstarch

4 large grapefruits, peeled and segmented

Preheat oven to 450°F. Cover baking sheet with foil. Divide beets into two clusters and place on the baking sheet. Sprinkle beets with the water. Roast 45 minutes or until beets are tender enough to be pierced with a fork. Cool. Rub off skins and slice thin.

Combine grapefruit juice, maple syrup, and vinegar in a bowl. Place cornstarch in a small saucepan and slowly whisk in grapefruit juice mixture until all cornstarch is dissolved.

Bring to a boil over medium heat, whisking frequently. Reduce heat to medium-low and cook 3 to 5 minutes, stirring often, until the sauce is glossy and thickened.

Place beets and grapefruit segments in a large bowl and toss. Transfer to a serving platter, drizzle with grapefruit glaze, and serve.

VARIATIONS

▶ Try golden beets in place of the red variety.

▶ Use raw honey in place of maple syrup.

▶ Top glaze with fresh chives or pea sprouts.

Soy Succotash

YIELD: 6 servings

PREPARATION TIME: 30 minutes

Fresh-frozen soybeans (edamame) stand in for the traditional lima beans in this sweet and nutty classic revisited.

2 teaspoons canola or grapeseed oil
½ cup chopped red bell pepper
¼ cup chopped yellow or green onions
2 cloves garlic, minced
2 cups frozen corn kernels
1½ cups frozen shelled edamame (soybeans)
3 tablespoons white wine or low-sodium vegetable broth
2 tablespoons chopped fresh parsley
1 tablespoon chopped fresh basil or 1 teaspoon dried basil
½ teaspoon salt or kelp powder
¼ teaspoon ground black pepper
Sprinkle soy lecithin granules

Heat oil in large nonstick skillet over medium heat. Add bell pepper, onion, and garlic. Cook 2 minutes, stirring frequently. Stir in corn, edamame, and wine or vegetable broth. Cook 4 minutes, stirring frequently. Remove pan from heat.

Stir in parsley, basil, salt or kelp powder, and pepper.

Transfer to a platter, sprinkle with soy lecithin granules, and serve warm, or serve cold as a salad over watercress.

··· VARIATIONS: ···

► Use yellow, green, or black bell pepper in place of red.
► Use 2 cups cubed summer squash in place of corn.
► To serve as a main dish, add 1 cup cubed plain or seasoned firm tofu or cooked tempeh.

MAIN DISHES

Black Bean and Walnut Burgers

YIELD: 6 servings

PREPARATION TIME: 20 minutes

The best bean for burgers has a smoky flavor and more omega-3s than other beans plus eight different free-radical-fighting phytonutrients.

2½ cups cooked black beans, divided

1 teaspoon ground cumin

2 teaspoons chili powder

¼ teaspoon cayenne pepper

½ cup cooked brown rice

¼ cup chopped walnuts

½ cup chopped red onion

Salt and pepper to taste

⅓ cup cornmeal

Chunky salsa or sliced orange for garnish

Puree 2 cups beans with cumin, chili powder, and cayenne pepper until smooth. Add rice, walnuts, onion, and remaining beans; mixture should be stiff but not dry. Add 2 tablespoons water to moisten, if necessary. Season to taste with salt and pepper. Cover and chill, if making ahead of time.

Divide mixture into six burgers. Dredge in cornmeal. Chill for 30 minutes (unless mixture has been prechilled).

Grease skillet with cooking spray. Cook burgers over medium heat for 4 minutes. Flip, and cook for an additional 4 minutes, or until heated through.

Garnish with salsa or sliced orange.

··· **VARIATIONS** ···

▶ Substitute red beans or black-eyed peas for black beans.

▶ Add 2 tablespoons ground flaxseeds for more omega-3s.

▶ Use peanuts in place of walnuts.

▶ Garnish with sprouted lentils.

Sizzlin' Seitan

YIELD: 6 to 8 servings

PREPARATION TIME: 20 minutes

Developed by vegetarian pacifist monks, and sometimes known as Buddha food, seitan is made from the protein portion of wheat and spares you calories and fat.

¼ cup olive oil

16 ounces seitan, sliced

2 medium red onions, cut into ½-inch dice (1 cup)

2 yellow bell peppers, cut into ½-inch dice (1 cup)

¼ cup peeled and minced fresh gingerroot

2 14-ounce cans light coconut milk

2 large mangoes, peeled and cut into ¾-inch cubes or use frozen, divided (2 cups)

1 cup unsweetened pineapple juice

2 tablespoons curry powder

1 teaspoon salt

¼ cup chopped chives for garnish

4 cups cooked brown rice

Heat oil in a large skillet over medium-high heat. Add seitan, and cook 1 to 2 minutes per side, or until lightly golden. Transfer to a plate, and set aside.

Reduce heat to medium. Add onion and bell peppers to skillet, and sauté 4 minutes or until softened. Add gingerroot, and sauté for 30 seconds or until fragrant. Stir in coconut milk, 1 cup mangoes, pineapple juice, curry powder, and seitan. Cover, and bring to a boil. Reduce heat to medium-low, and simmer 5 minutes. Uncover, and simmer for 10 more minutes, or until thickened, stirring occasionally.

Top with remaining mango cubes and chives. Serve over rice.

··· **VARIATIONS** ···

► Use tempeh Instead of seitan.
► Try grapeseed oil in place of olive oil.
► Use green bell peppers not yellow.
► Substitute quinoa, barley, or lentils for rice.
► Peaches can replace mangoes.

Chard and Barley Stew

YIELD: 6 servings

PREPARATION TIME: 1 hour

No meat, no potatoes, but plenty of fiber and phytochemicals.

2 tablespoons olive oil

1¼ pounds Swiss chard, leaves and
stems separated and diced

2 medium leeks, halved and sliced

3 medium carrots, peeled and sliced

2 stalks celery, sliced

Pinch ground nutmeg

2 cups low-sodium vegetable broth

1 cup medium pearled barley

1 cup water

1 cup frozen lima beans

Heat oil in large stockpot over medium-high heat. Stir in chard stems, leeks, carrots, celery, and nutmeg. Cook 6 to 7 minutes until vegetables release juices but still retain their color. Add broth, barley, and water. Cover, and bring to a boil. Reduce heat and simmer, covered, for 45 minutes, stirring occasionally. Add lima beans and chard leaves. Simmer for 10 more minutes.

··· **VARIATIONS** ···

▶ Use parsnips in place of carrots.

▶ Use jicama or water chestnuts in place of celery.

▶ Use frozen edamame or peas in place of limas.

▶ Garnish with cornbread croutons or broccoli sprouts.

Better Red Risotto

YIELD: 6 servings

PREPARATION TIME: 35 minutes

Radicchio and tomatoes are the "red" antioxidants in this creamy risotto.

3 cups low-sodium vegetable broth
3 cups water
2 tablespoons olive oil, divided
1 medium red onion, chopped
2 small heads radicchio, cored and
    cut into strips
1½ cups arborio rice
1 teaspoon sugar
⅔ cup dry red wine

4 small plum tomatoes, seeded and
    coarsely chopped
4 ounces smoked mozzarella or
    4 ounces firm nondairy cheese,
    grated
½ cup chopped fresh parsley
¼ cup grated Parmesan cheese (or
    nondairy equivalent)
Salt and pepper to taste

Place broth and water in large glass measuring cup. Heat in the microwave until boiling.

Heat 1 tablespoon oil in heavy skillet over medium heat. Add onion, and cook 5 minutes, stirring, until golden. Add radicchio, and cook for 4 minutes or until wilted. Stir in the rice and sugar; cook for 2 minutes, while stirring. Add wine, and cook until wine is almost absorbed. Add ½ cup hot broth mixture, and cook again until almost absorbed. Continue gradually adding broth, allowing rice to absorb liquid, about 10 minutes. Stir in tomatoes, and cook 2 to 3 minutes longer. Remove from heat, and stir in remaining oil and mozzarella (or the nondairy substitute). Add the parsley and Parmesan or Parmesan substitute. Season as needed with salt and pepper.

··· **VARIATIONS** ···

► Substitute arugula for radicchio.
► Use short-grain brown rice in place of arborio.
► Add ½ cup to 1 cup sautéed mushrooms.
► Top with a dab of Mustard Greens Pesto (page 142).

DIY Thai Curry (Raw)

YIELD: 4 servings

PREPARATION TIME: 20 minutes

Raw and rich in enzymes for better digestion.

1½-inch piece peeled fresh
    gingerroot
1 cup soaked peanuts, drained
    (soak ⅔ cup peanuts in water for
    8 hours)
1 cup shredded young coconut meat
½ cup coconut water
1 tablespoon raw almond butter
2 teaspoons sea salt or to taste
1 clove garlic, pressed
1 teaspoon turmeric

1 teaspoon curry powder
Juice of 1 orange
1 Thai chili
¼ head cauliflower, diced
1 small carrot, shredded
¼ head red cabbage, shredded
½ cucumber, peeled and cut into
    half-moons
Basil leaves for garnish
Mung bean sprouts for garnish

To prepare sauce, finely grate the gingerroot to extract juice. Blend ginger juice, peanuts, coconut meat, coconut water, almond butter, salt, garlic, turmeric, curry powder, and orange juice in blender until smooth. Add the Thai chili to taste.

Place cauliflower, carrot, cabbage, and cucumber in bowl. Pour sauce over vegetables. Garnish with basil and bean sprouts.

··· **VARIATIONS** ···

► Substitute broccoliflower for cauliflower.
► Use cashew butter in place of almond butter.
► Omit chili for a less spicy dish.
► Add ¼ cup diced red bell pepper.

No-Fry Fritters

YIELD: 6 servings

PREPARATION TIME: 25 minutes

With this dish, there is no unsafe frying and no spattering oil. These fritters crisp up just fine in your oven. Quinoa complements the tender cauliflower.

½ cup quinoa

1 cup water

½ teaspoon salt

1 cup cauliflower florets

¼ cup grated Parmesan cheese

2 large eggs

2 tablespoons chopped flat-leaf parsley

2 tablespoons bread crumbs

¼ teaspoon black pepper

Basil-and-garlic-flavored tomato sauce (store-bought)

Coat a baking sheet with cooking spray and set aside. Heat a saucepan over high heat. Add quinoa and toast 3 minutes, or until it begins to pop, stirring constantly. Add water and salt, and bring to a boil. Cover, and lower heat to medium-low, and let simmer 10 minutes or until water is absorbed. Cool.

Meantime, cook cauliflower in boiling water for 8 minutes. Drain, and break into small pieces.

Preheat oven to 450°F. Mix quinoa, cauliflower, Parmesan, eggs, parsley, bread crumbs, and pepper in a large bowl (mixture will be moist and loose). Shape into 3-inch patties. Arrange on prepared baking sheet, and bake for 20 minutes, or until fritters are golden brown.

Serve with tomato sauce.

··· **VARIATIONS** ···

► Substitute amaranth for quinoa.

► Add 2 tablespoons chopped black olives.

► Top with light-colored miso (mild) or dark-colored miso (pungent).

Hijiki Stir-Fry

YIELD: 4 servings

PREPARATION TIME: 20 minutes

*There are vegetables from the land and
the sea in this skillet-to-table dish.*

½ cup hijiki (dried seaweed)

1 tablespoon sesame oil

2 cloves garlic, minced

1 tablespoon peeled and grated
fresh gingerroot

½ onion, chopped

½ cup chopped celery

1 cup chopped carrots

1 cup broccoli florets, chopped
cabbage, or both

Juice of ½ lemon

1 tablespoon low-sodium soy sauce
or tamari

¼ cup filtered water

1 teaspoon maple syrup

1 tablespoon mirin (or sweet white
wine)

1 tablespoon white sesame seeds for
garnish

Rinse and soak the hijiki for 15 minutes in warm water to cover.

Heat sesame oil in frying pan or wok. Add garlic, gingerroot, and onion. Sauté until the onions are translucent (about 2 minutes). Add the hijiki, celery, carrots, broccoli, and cabbage, and continue to sauté.

Mix the lemon juice, soy sauce or tamari, water, maple syrup, and mirin, and add them to the vegetables. Cover, and let simmer for 5 minutes.

Spoon into serving dish. Garnish with sesame seeds, and serve.

··· **VARIATIONS** ···

▶ Add 1 cup sautéed tofu.

▶ Double quantity, and serve as a main dish.

▶ Use summer squash in place of celery.

▶ Use cauliflower in place of broccoli.

▶ Use white grape juice in place of wine.

▶ Add ½ cup red bell pepper strips in place of ½ cup carrots.

▶ Use flaxseeds in place of sesame seeds.

Meatless Cacciatore

YIELD: 6 servings

PREPARATION TIME: 1 hour, 10 minutes

Tofu replaces beef in this five-vegetable stew without meat.

2 tablespoons olive oil

2 medium-size onions, coarsely chopped (about 2 cups)

1 large green or red pepper, cut into 1½-inch strips

3 large cloves garlic, minced (1 tablespoon)

1 28-ounce can diced tomatoes

2 8-ounce bags baby carrots, halved diagonally

1 8-ounce package Italian-flavored baked tofu, cut into cubes

1 tablespoon rubbed dried sage

1 bay leaf

Salt and pepper to taste

12 ounces whole grain pasta

Heat olive oil in large pot over medium heat. Add onions and pepper, and cook 5 to 7 minutes, or until softened, stirring often. Add garlic, and cook 1 minute more or until fragrant. Stir in tomatoes, carrots, tofu, sage, and bay leaf. Season with salt and pepper. Cover, reduce heat to medium-low, and simmer about 1 hour, or until carrots are tender. Remove bay leaf.

After the cacciatore has simmered about 45 minutes, cook pasta according to package directions. Serve cacciatore over the prepared pasta.

··· VARIATIONS ···

► Substitute steamed quinoa or wild rice for pasta.

► Stir in ½ cup to 1 cup sea vegetables for more protein and minerals, or add 1 cup of plain or spicy tofu.

Parsnip-Ginger Curry

YIELD: 4 servings

PREPARATION TIME: 25 minutes

Parsnips, the spud stand-in, are lower in calories and higher in fiber and even more nutritious coupled with curry and ginger.

3 tablespoons peanut oil

2 cloves garlic, finely chopped

1-inch piece fresh gingerroot, peeled and finely grated

2 red chilies, seeded and finely sliced

1 lemongrass stem, finely sliced

2 kaffir lime leaves, finely shredded (optional)

1 large onion, diced

⅓ cup tomato paste

1 13.5-ounce can unsweetened coconut milk

2 pounds parsnips, peeled and cut into ¾-inch cubes

1 small bunch cilantro, stems intact, washed well, divided

3 tablespoons low-sodium soy sauce

Salt to taste

1 teaspoon lime juice

2 tablespoons chopped green or black olives for garnish

Heat oil over medium heat in a deep saucepan, add garlic, ginger, chilies, lemongrass, kaffir lime leaves (optional), and onion. Sauté until they begin to caramelize, about 10 minutes. Add tomato paste, stirring well for another 30 seconds. Add coconut milk and parsnips. Add water to cover, and bring to a boil. Remove and reserve leaves from cilantro; then chop stems as fine as you can and add to curry. Bring curry to a simmer, cover pot, and cook until parsnips can easily be pierced by fork. Mix in the soy sauce, add salt to taste, and then remove from heat.

Just before serving, stir in cilantro leaves and lime juice. Garnish with chopped green or black olives.

··· **VARIATIONS** ··

▶ Substitute 1 tablespoon fresh lemon zest for lemongrass.

▶ Use rice milk in place of coconut milk.

Purple Potato Colcannon

YIELD: 6 servings

PREPARATION TIME: 35 minutes

This is the twenty-first-century version (shiitakes added) of an Irish country dish. If you can't find the traditional colcannon ingredient— purple potatoes—then substitute Yukon gold or russet potatoes.

1 pound purple potatoes

½ pound kale, tough stems removed

½ pound broccoli

2 to 3 tablespoons olive oil

10 ounces shiitake mushrooms, sliced (about 3 cups)

3 cloves garlic, chopped (about 1 tablespoon)

Salt and pepper to taste

1 cup unsweetened rice milk, warmed

Place potatoes in large pot, and cover with water. Bring to a boil, reduce heat to medium, and simmer 15 to 20 minutes. Drain, and return to pot. Heat potatoes over medium heat for 2 minutes to steam off excess water, and set aside.

Meanwhile, bring a large pot of salted water to a boil. Add kale and broccoli; cook 5 minutes. Drain, and set aside.

Heat oil in a large skillet over medium heat. Add mushrooms and garlic, and sauté 5 to 7 minutes, or until mushrooms are soft and all liquid has evaporated. Stir in kale and broccoli, and cook for an additional minute or until hot. Season with salt and pepper.

Mash rice milk into potatoes until soft but still chunky. Fold in kale mixture, and serve.

VARIATIONS

▶ Use white and red cabbage in place of kale and broccoli.

▶ Use any other mushroom in place of shiitake.

▶ Use soy or dairy milk in place of rice milk.

Hijiki-Shiitake Sloppy Joes

YIELD: 4 servings

PREPARATION TIME: 30 minutes

*Shiitakes are a source of the compound lentian, which
maximizes immunity throughout the body; it's even more
powerful paired with the sea vegetable hijiki.*

1½ ounces hijiki

5 large or 10 small shiitake
   mushrooms

2 tablespoons extra-virgin olive oil

2 medium carrots, peeled and
   shredded

1 cup cooked soybeans or pinto
   beans

1 cup low-sodium vegetable broth

1 tablespoon honey

¼ cup low-sodium soy sauce

1 cup cooked tempeh, tofu, seitan, or
   cubed cheese

Soak hijiki in cold water to cover, and soak shiitake mushrooms in hot
water; soak each for 10 minutes. Drain mushrooms (keeping the soaking
water), and slice.

Heat olive oil in a large skillet over medium-high heat. Drain hijiki,
and place in skillet, stirring. Add carrots and mushrooms, stirring. Add
soybeans, mushroom soaking water, vegetable broth, honey, and soy
sauce. Turn heat to medium-low, and cook for abut 10 minutes, until
carrots are tender. Stir in tempeh, tofu, seitan, or cubed cheese. Adjust
seasoning. Add more water, if needed, for a thick sloppy Joe.

··· **VARIATIONS** ···

▶ For a side dish, omit the final ingredient.

▶ Substitute cremini, enoki, or another mushroom for shiitakes.

▶ Use arame in place of hijiki.

▶ Add ½ cup sliced green olives.

▶ Add ¼ cup sautéed red bell peppers for color and crunch.

Multivitamin Moussaka

YIELD: 6 servings

PREPARATION TIME: 1½ hours

Potatoes to tomatoes and plenty of nutrients in this assembled-like-lasagna dish.

2 large russet potatoes, peeled and cut into large dice

2 garlic cloves, peeled

¼ cup olive oil, divided

¼ cup chopped green or yellow onions

1 tablespoon dried oregano

2 cups chopped canned or fresh tomatoes with juice

⅓ cup green lentils

1 small bay leaf

½ cinnamon stick

Salt and pepper (or kelp powder or dulse), to taste

1 medium eggplant, sliced

1 small zucchini, sliced

1 large tomato, thinly sliced

Cook potatoes and garlic in boiling salted water for 10 minutes until soft; reserve liquid. Mash potatoes with olive oil, reserving 1 tablespoon, and add 1 cup of reserved cooking liquid to the potato-garlic mixture.

Heat remaining olive oil in saucepan over medium heat. Add onion and oregano, and sauté for 5 minutes. Add tomatoes, lentils, bay leaf, cinnamon stick, and about a cup of the reserved potato cooking water. Cover, reduce heat to medium-low, and simmer until lentils are tender. Remove bay leaf and cinnamon stick. Pulse lentil mixture briefly in blender until slightly chunky. Season with salt and pepper (or kelp powder or dulse).

Place eggplant slices on paper-towel-lined baking sheet, and sprinkle with salt. Let stand 15 minutes; rinse and pat dry.

Preheat oven to 350°F, and oil a deep 13″ × 9″ baking dish. Spoon one-third of the lentil mixture into dish, followed by the zucchini and tomato slices. Spoon on another third of the lentil mixture, and top with half the potatoes. Top with eggplant and the rest of the lentil mixture. Add remaining potatoes. Bake 1 hour until top is completely browned.

▶ Add ½ cup tofu cut into matchstick slivers on top of the first lentil-mixture layer.

▶ In place of zucchini, use ¼ cup cooked sea vegetables such as arame or hijiki.

▶ Use leeks in place of onion.

▶ Sprinkle with lentil sprouts before serving.

Wheat Meat Meatballs

YIELD: 6 servings

PREPARATION TIME: 1 hour

Seitan, or "wheat meat," which takes on the flavor of the herbs and spices or sauces it is cooked with, can be diced, sliced, or ground into patties and stir-fried, boiled, broiled, or, as here, baked.

16-ounce package seitan (Note: seitan is slightly more perishable than tofu, so check the expiration date before buying)

1½ cup pecans

½ cup whole wheat bread crumbs

¼ cup chopped fresh parsley

¼ cup chopped fresh basil

3 tablespoons olive oil, divided

3 cloves garlic, minced

1 teaspoon low-sodium soy sauce

¼ teaspoon dried oregano

1 small egg

Preheat oven to 400°F. Lightly grease a cookie sheet.

Blend seitan in food processor until crumbly. Add pecans and pulse. Place in bowl, and stir in bread crumbs, herbs, 1 teaspoon oil, garlic, soy sauce, and oregano. Add egg to mixture. Shape mixture into 12 to 18 meatballs. Place on baking sheet, and brush with remaining oil.

Bake 20 minutes, turning once. Balls should be crispy brown.

Serve over whole-grain noodles or pasta or steamed rice. Top with tomato or mushroom sauce.

VARIATIONS

▶ Substitute tempeh for seitan.

▶ Use cilantro in place of parsley.

▶ Add ¼ cup finely chopped green or black olives to seitan mixture.

▶ Add 1 tablespoon flaxseed meal or soy lecithin granules to boost antioxidants.

Immunity Meatloaf

YIELD: 4 to 6 servings

PREPARATION TIME: 45 minutes

Serve warm today, cold tomorrow; it's nourishing both ways.

1 cup cooked brown rice
½ cup finely chopped walnuts
½ cup diced mushrooms
1 small onion, finely chopped
¼ cup finely chopped bell pepper
1 large carrot, shredded
½ cup wheat germ or oat bran
½ cup quick-cooking oats

¼ teaspoon each dried marjoram, sage, and thyme
1 teaspoon low-sodium soy sauce or tamari
1 teaspoon Dijon-style mustard
¼ cup natural ketchup or barbecue sauce

Preheat oven to 350°F. Combine all ingredients except ketchup or barbecue sauce. Mix well. Pat mixture into a well-greased loaf pan, and spread on ketchup or barbecue sauce. Bake 50 minutes, and let stand 10 minutes before serving.

··· **VARIATIONS** ···

▶ Substitute cooked bulgur or kasha for brown rice.
▶ Add 1 teaspoon kelp or dulse powder.
▶ Use roasted unsalted peanuts in place of walnuts.
▶ Replace bell pepper with Italian pepper or a firm tomato.
▶ Replace half of the wheat germ with flaxseeds.

Spicy Tofu Minute Steaks

YIELD: 4 servings

PREPARATION TIME: 30 minutes or less

Anti-cancer fast food.

4 teaspoons sesame seeds, white or black, for garnish

4 strips orange zest in thin slivers, divided

1 cup fresh-squeezed orange juice

2 tablespoons balsamic vinegar

1 tablespoon toasted sesame oil

1 tablespoon low-sodium soy sauce or tamari

2 tablespoons brown sugar

½ teaspoon five-spice powder

2 packages firm tofu (about 2 pounds), drained and sliced lengthwise into "steaks"

2 green onions, chopped diagonally, for garnish

Toast sesame seeds for 5 minutes in a dry skillet, shaking until they are fragrant.

Plunge zest in boiling water, simmer 2 minutes, and then drain.

Bring juice, vinegar, sesame oil, soy sauce, brown sugar, five-spice powder, and half of the zest to a boil in a large skillet over medium heat. Add tofu, reduce heat to medium-low, and simmer for about 8 minutes until all liquid is gone. Cook an additional 3 minutes, shaking pan, until steaks are browned and glazed.

Garnish with green onions, the rest of the zest, and sesame seeds.

VARIATIONS

► Substitute a pinch of cinnamon and another pinch of fennel, plus a few grinds of black pepper, for the five-spice powder (cinnamon, fennel, black pepper, cloves, and star anise).

► Add ½ cup of cooked sea vegetables to the dish before serving.

► Use sunflower oil in place of sesame oil.

► Add a pinch of cayenne pepper to enhance flavors.

► Instead of green onions, garnish with sprouts and sliced kiwi or star fruit.

Blackened Tempeh

YIELD: 4 servings

PREPARATION TIME: 30 minutes

Enzymes created during the fermentation of tempeh make this
complete protein food easier to digest than meat or poultry.

½ cup instant black bean mix
(prepackaged fully cooked black
beans ready to be reconstituted)
¾ cup hot water
2 8-ounce pieces tempeh
2 tablespoons Cajun spice mix

2 tablespoons low-sodium soy sauce
or tamari
1 teaspoon stevia or 2 tablespoons
natural sugar (such as Sucanat)
2 tablespoons canola or grapeseed
cooking oil

In a bowl, combine bean mix and hot water. Blend well, and set aside.

Slice each length of tempeh in half, and use a sharp knife to make a
slit along the side. Open and fill with ¼ cup of the bean mix. Press each
piece closed, and set aside.

In a small bowl, combine Cajun spice mix with 2 tablespoons water,
soy sauce or tamari, and sweetener. Brush this mixture on both sides of
the stuffed tempeh.

Heat oil in large skillet, and sauté the stuffed tempeh on both sides
until browned. Place prepared tempeh in baking dish, cover, and bake for
10 to 15 minutes.

Serve plain or with tomato sauce.

··· **VARIATIONS** ···

► Stuff with steamed millet or quinoa instead of black bean mix.
► Top with grated mozzarella or soy mozzarella cheese before baking.
► Sprinkle with cooked dulse, hijiki, or other sea vegetable before
serving.

Rosemary and Thyme Frittata

YIELD: 4 to 6 servings

PREPARATION TIME: 45 minutes

*Healthier than fritters and tasty hot or cold under
a mild miso sauce or a little salsa.*

2 tablespoons extra-virgin olive oil, divided

2 small leeks, cleaned and thinly sliced

6 large eggs

1 cup tofu or ricotta cheese

¼ cup pitted and finely chopped green olives

3 tablespoons pine nuts, lightly toasted

2 tablespoons chopped flat-leaf parsley

2 teaspoons chopped fresh thyme

½ teaspoon chopped fresh rosemary

½ teaspoon salt

Set rack in the middle of the oven, and preheat to 400°F.

Heat 1 tablespoon of oil in a large ovenproof skillet over medium-high heat. Add leeks and cook, stirring until leeks are soft and lightly browned.

In a medium bowl, combine eggs, tofu (or ricotta), olives, pine nuts, the three herbs and salt. Beat lightly with a fork until just combined. Use a rubber spatula to add the leeks to the egg mixture. Stir to combine, and wipe out the skillet.

Reheat skillet, and add remaining oil. Pour in egg mixture, and place skillet in oven. Bake until eggs are barely set, about 20 minutes.

Transfer pan from oven to broiler (about 4 inches from heat source). Broil until golden brown; watch carefully.

Serve hot or cold.

Summer-Squash Pasta with Summer Herbs

YIELD: 4 servings

PREPARATION TIME: 30 minutes

Vegetables married with a grain pasta and fortified with herbs and cheese to make a holistic whole-meal summer salad.

2 small zucchini, shaved into ribbons (stop at seeds)

2 small yellow squash, shaved into ribbons (stop at seeds)

1 tablespoon extra-virgin olive oil

¼ teaspoon grated lemon zest

1 teaspoon fresh-squeezed lemon juice

¼ teaspoon salt or kelp or dulse powder

Pinch black pepper

1 garlic clove, minced

¼ cup thinly sliced fresh basil

1 teaspoon chopped fresh oregano or ½ teaspoon dried

2 cups cooked whole wheat pasta

Freshly grated Parmesan cheese (or a vegan alternative) for garnish

Place zucchini and summer squash in a bowl.

Combine oil, lemon zest, lemon juice, salt (or kelp or dulse), pepper, and garlic in a small bowl. Stir with a whisk, and drizzle over vegetable ribbons. Sprinkle with basil and oregano, and toss. Fold in cooked pasta, and sprinkle with cheese. Serve at room temperature or chill before serving.

··· **VARIATION** ···

► Sprinkle with toasted flaxseeds or broccoli sprouts.

Hoppin' John Burgers

YIELD: 6 servings

PREPARATION TIME: 30 minutes

This spicy, meatless Southern-inspired lunch or dinner entree uses corn in place of the rice in a traditional Hoppin' John recipe.

3 cups cooked black-eyed peas

2 cups fresh or frozen corn kernels

1 tablespoon canola or grapeseed oil, divided

1 tablespoon mashed garlic

1 jalapeño pepper, seeded and minced, or ¼ cup chopped canned green chilies

¼ teaspoon cumin

½ cup minced green onions

¼ teaspoon minced cilantro

½ teaspoon salt or kelp powder

Mash black-eyed peas coarsely with mixer or food processor, and set aside.

Puree fresh or slightly defrosted frozen corn in blender or food processor.

Heat half the oil in a large skillet, and add garlic, pepper (or chilies), and cumin. Sauté 2 minutes, and add corn. Reduce heat to low, and cook 3 minutes, stirring constantly.

Mix mashed peas, corn mixture, green onions, cilantro, and salt or kelp. Cool.

Wet hands and form mixture into six patties, each about 3 inches in diameter.

Reoil the skillet with remaining oil. Heat to medium-hot, and cook burgers 5 minutes on each side or until golden crisp and thoroughly cooked.

Serve hot over rice or inside whole-grain buns, topped with olive tapenade or Moroccan "Caviar" (see page 135). Sprinkle with pea shoots or lentil sprouts.

··· **VARIATIONS** ···

▶ Substitute black beans for black-eyed peas.

▶ Substitute brown rice for corn.

▶ Use ¼ cup mashed black or green olives in place of jalapeños for a less spicy version.

▶ Sprinkle with soy lecithin granules before serving.

DESSERTS

Beta-Glucan Oatmeal Cookies

MAKES: 48 cookies

PREPARATION TIME: 30 minutes

Beta-glucan, the immune-boosting fiber in oats, is abundant in these egg-and-butter-free, healthier-than-most cookies.

1½ cups whole wheat pastry flour
½ cup unbleached white flour
2 teaspoons baking powder
½ teaspoon salt
1 cup sugar, preferably organic (e.g., Sucanat, Florida Crystals)
1¼ cups quick-cooking (not instant) rolled oats

1 to 2 teaspoons cinnamon
1 cup soft tofu
1 cup vanilla yogurt
½ teaspoon vanilla extract
¼ cup cold-pressed grapeseed or canola oil
1 cup diced figs or dates

Preheat oven to 350°F. Sift flours with the baking powder, salt, and sugar. Stir in oats and cinnamon. In a separate bowl, beat tofu with yogurt, vanilla, and oil. Combine two mixtures; then fold in dried fruits and mix well.

On a greased cookie sheet, drop batter by the teaspoonful, leaving an inch between each cookie. Press each with the back of a fork. Bake for 15 to 17 minutes until firm and slightly browned. Cool on a rack.

··· VARIATIONS ···

▶ Add ¼ cup of any raw nut.
▶ Add 2 tablespoons flaxseeds.
▶ Use raisins in place of figs or dates.
▶ Use buttermilk in place of yogurt.

Probiotic Parfait

YIELD: 6 to 8 servings

PREPARATION TIME: 15 minutes, plus 1 hour freezing time

Ice cream one better—good bacteria for the gut and berry antioxidants for the brain, without the sugar and fat.

2 cups vanilla yogurt
½ cup milk or soy half-and-half
1 teaspoon stevia

1 10-ounce package frozen raspberries, thawed
Fresh raspberries or fresh mint for garnish (optional)

Combine first three ingredients in large bowl. Place thawed raspberries in blender, and process until smooth. Add puree to yogurt mixture. Pour into a freezer-safe container. Cover and freeze for at least 1 hour. Garnish with fresh berries or mint.

VARIATIONS

► Stir in 2 tablespoons flaxseeds.
► Use strawberries in place of raspberries.
► Add a handful of soaked dried goji berries as a garnish, or fold unsoaked berries into the mixture for crunch.
► Use raw honey in place of stevia.

Pie in a Glass 1

YIELD: 2 servings

PREPARATION TIME: 10 minutes

Immunity-boosting but dairy- and sugar-free treat.

2 pitted dates soaked in hot water
  to cover until soft, then drained
½ cup fresh or canned pineapple
  chunks
½ cup fresh strawberries, hulled, or
  frozen strawberries, thawed

4 ounces soft silken tofu, drained
1 medium-size ripe banana, peeled,
  cut into chunks, and frozen
1 cup applesauce, unsweetened, or
  1 cup pureed apples

In a blender, combine dates, pineapple, strawberries, and tofu; process until smooth. Add banana and applesauce or puree, and blend until thick and smooth.

Pour into two glasses, and serve immediately.

Pie in a Glass 2

YIELD: 2 servings

PREPARATION TIME: 10 minutes

No dairy, no sugar, but four-fruit fortified.

½ medium-size ripe cantaloupe, seeded, rind removed, and cut into chunks
½ cup orange juice, fresh-squeezed or from concentrate
Juice of 2 limes

1 medium-size ripe banana, peeled, cut into chunks, and frozen
Fresh mint leaves for garnish (optional)

Place cantaloupe in blender. Add orange juice, lime juice, and banana. Blend until thick and creamy.

Pour into two glasses, and garnish with mint leaves. Serve at once.

··· VARIATIONS ···

► Add 1 cup soft tofu.
► Add ¼ cup acai berries, goji berries, or blueberries.
► Garnish with crushed pistachios or cashews.

Dried-Fruit Truffles

YIELD: 36 truffles

PREPARATION TIME: 15 minutes, including chilling time

*Guilt-free sweet that is rich in bone-building
calcium, magnesium, zinc, plus fiber.*

1½ cups pitted dates, soaked in hot water to cover until soft

2 cups raw cashews

½ cup soy milk or other dairy-free milk

Drain dates, and set aside.

Process cashews in blender or food processor until finely ground. Reserve ½ cup, and set aside. Add dates to remaining cashews, and process till well blended. Add enough soy milk to hold mixture together. Roll mixture into 1-inch balls between your palms. Roll in the reserved cashews, and place on platter or baking sheet. Cover and refrigerate until ready to serve. This dessert will keep for as long as two weeks if tightly covered in refrigerator.

VARIATIONS

▶ Use dried figs in place of dates.

▶ Use dairy milk in place of soy.

▶ Substitute walnuts for cashews.

▶ Add grated orange or lemon zest.

Health Halvah

YIELD: 24 pieces

PREPARATION TIME: 15 minutes, plus 1 hour chilling time

*This halvah is raw and rich in both enzymes
and cholesterol-lowering lignans.*

1½ cups almonds
½ cup raw tahini
1 teaspoon vanilla extract
3 tablespoons honey or rice syrup

1 tablespoon soy lecithin granules
1 tablespoon plus 1 teaspoon dark
   cocoa powder

Place almonds in food processor (or nut mill) and process until finely ground. Add tahini, vanilla, honey, and lecithin, and process well. Put half the mixture in a bowl, and set aside. Add cocoa to the remaining mix and process. Press plain mixture into pan until it is ¼ inch thick. Press the chocolate mixture over the plain mixture to create a ½-inch-thick, two-colored slab. Chill for an hour (or more). Cut into bite-sized pieces, and roll into balls.

··· **VARIATIONS** ···

► Substitute pecans for half the almonds.
► Add almond extract in place of vanilla.
► Add a sprinkle of ground red pepper to enhance flavors.
► Add 1 teaspoon lemon zest instead of vanilla.
► Use carob powder in place of cocoa powder.

Bellini Brownies

YIELD: 16 squares

PREPARATION TIME: 45 minutes

Better brownies—low in sugar, dairy free, and fruit enhanced.

¾ cup unbleached flour
¼ cup unsweetened cocoa powder
⅛ teaspoon baking powder
⅛ teaspoon baking soda
⅛ teaspoon salt
1 large fresh peach, pitted, peeled, and sliced

¼ cup dairy-free chocolate chips (or regular chips)
¼ cup grapeseed or canola oil
½ cup natural sugar or honey
½ cup plain soy milk
2 tablespoons flaxseed meal
1 teaspoon vanilla extract

Preheat oven to 350°F. Grease a 9-inch square baking pan.

Whisk the flour, cocoa powder, baking powder, baking soda, and salt in a large bowl.

Puree all but three slices of peaches, and set aside.

Melt chips with oil in a double boiler, stirring constantly. Remove from heat, and fold in peach puree and sugar or honey. Combine soy milk, flaxseed, and vanilla in a measuring cup, and fold into chocolate mixture. Fold chocolate mixture into flour mixture, and then pour into the prepared pan. Top with the remaining peach slices, and bake 20 to 25 minutes, until a toothpick inserted in the middle comes out clean. Cool in the pan on a wire rack before cutting into 16 squares.

··· **VARIATIONS** ···

► Substitute apricots for peaches.
► Add 1 tablespoon of soy lecithin granules with the flour and powders.
► Bake in a round pan, and cut into pie-shaped wedges.

Munch-and-Crunch Walnuts

YIELD: 1 cup

PREPARATION TIME: 20 minutes

Gotta snack? Get some omega-3s while you're at it.

1 cup coarsely chopped walnuts
1 teaspoon unsalted butter, melted
3 tablespoons honey, warmed

Sea salt or kosher salt
Pinch of cayenne pepper

Preheat oven to 350°F. Grease a pie plate or baking dish.

Place nuts on prepared dish and drizzle evenly with butter and honey. Roast until golden brown, stirring every few minutes. Transfer nuts to a plate, season with salt and cayenne, and let cool.

Nuts will keep for a month in an airtight container. Use as a sweet snack, as a dessert topping, or atop breakfast pancakes and waffles.

VARIATIONS

▶ Substitute peanuts for walnuts or use ½ cup of each.
▶ Sprinkle with sesame seeds before roasting.
▶ Omit cayenne and use kelp powder.

Papaya Pudding Smoothie

YIELD: 2 servings

PREPARATION TIME: 10 minutes

Sweet and creamy and beta-carotene rich but dairy and sugar free

1 cup peeled, cubed papaya

1 large banana, peeled

2 to 3 figs or pitted prunes

1 teaspoon soy lecithin granules

Place papaya in blender jar, and process briefly. Add banana, and process again. Add dried fruit and soy lecithin granules, and process until smooth.

Serve chilled in dessert cups, or spoon over yogurt.

VARIATIONS

▶ Use mango in place of papaya.

▶ Substitute dates for figs or prunes.

▶ Sprinkle with cinnamon or pumpkin pie spice before serving.

Pinot Noir Pears

YIELD: 3 servings

PREPARATION TIME: 20 minutes

Pear melba, nutritionally enhanced with dark chocolate and dairy-free ice cream.

2 cups medium-bodied red wine such as Pinot Noir
¼ cup sugar or ¼ teaspoon liquid stevia
1 tablespoon honey
1 stick cinnamon
2 whole cloves

3 Bosc pears, peeled, cored, and halved
Vanilla soy or dairy ice cream
1 ounce dark chocolate, shaved or finely chopped
1 tablespoon finely grated orange zest

Combine wine, sugar (or stevia), honey, cinnamon, and cloves in a large pot, and bring to a boil. Drop three pear halves in liquid, reduce heat to medium, and simmer for 10 minutes or until pears are tender. Remove fruit from cooking liquid, and repeat with remaining fruit. Strain the poaching liquid, and pour over the pears. Cool, cover, and refrigerate until ready to serve.

To serve, place a pear half in a dessert dish or cup, add a scoop of ice cream, and drizzle with poaching liquid. Top with chocolate and orange zest.

VARIATIONS

▶ Substitute another variety of pear such as the Comice, Bartlett, or Anjou.
▶ Substitute a thick yogurt such as Greek yogurt in place of ice cream to lower calories and fat.
▶ Sprinkle with toasted pistachios in place of orange zest.

Chocolate Tofousse

YIELD: 4 servings

PREPARATION TIME: 20 minutes, plus 2 hours chilling time

*This dessert is low fat, low cholesterol, and phytonu-
trient dense, but free of dairy and scant on sugar.*

5 ounces dark organic chocolate

3 tablespoons raw sugar (such as
Sucanat) or 2 teaspoons stevia

8 ounces extra-firm tofu

1 tablespoon flaxseeds

3 egg whites at room temperature

Chocolate curls for garnish

Melt chocolate and sugar (or stevia) together in double boiler, stirring
constantly. Remove from heat and cool. Puree the mixture with tofu,
stopping to scrape sides of blender jar with a rubber spatula. Put
chocolate-tofu mixture in a bowl, and stir in flaxseeds.

In a separate bowl, beat egg whites until almost stiff. Use spatula
to fold egg whites into chocolate-tofu mixture a little at a time, being
careful not to overmix. Refrigerate for at least 2 hours or longer for best
flavor.

Before serving, garnish with chocolate curls made with a vegetable
peeler.

VARIATIONS

► Stir in 1 teaspoon orange zest for orange-flavored Tofousse.
► Stir in ¼ cup crushed nuts for crunch.

Chai Rice Pudding

YIELD: 4 servings

PREPARATION TIME: 45 minutes

*Smack your lips and strengthen your arteries
with this fat- and dairy-free dessert.*

1 cup water

1½ cups unsweetened soy milk or
low-fat milk, divided

2 black chai tea bags

½ cup short-grain rice

¼ cup natural brown sugar

Pinch salt

1 small apple, cored and diced (don't
peel if organic)

¼ cup raisins

Whipped tofu for garnish

Cinnamon for garnish

Bring water and ½ cup soy milk to a boil in a large saucepan. Remove from heat, and add tea bags. Cover and steep 5 minutes. Remove tea bags, squeezing out any liquid. Stir rice, sugar, and salt into tea mixture, and bring to a boil over medium heat. Reduce heat, cover, and simmer for 10 minutes. Add remaining soy milk or milk, and simmer uncovered until rice is soft, about 15 to 20 minutes. Stir in apples and raisins. Remove from heat, cover, and let sit for 10 minutes.

Serve hot or cold. Garnish with whipped tofu and a sprinkle of cinnamon.

VARIATIONS

▶ Substitute other dried fruit (dates, figs, dried blueberries, or dried cherries) for raisins.

▶ Use ¼ cup honey in place of sugar.

▶ Sprinkle finished pudding with a mixture of soy lecithin granules and flaxseeds.

Drop-Outs

YIELD: 18 cookies

PREPARATION TIME: 20 minutes, plus drying time

Raw enzyme-rich (but dairy-free) fruit-and-nut drop cookies.

1 cup sunflower seeds
¼ cup pine nuts
1 teaspoon flaxseed meal
Pinch sea salt

6 to 8 dates, pitted and chopped
1 to 2 tablespoons orange or apple
juice

Grind the sunflower seeds and pine nuts in a nut mill or coffee grinder to make nut meal.

Put nut meal into food processor with flaxseed meal and salt, and add dates one at a time, until a dough begins to form. Taste for sweetness, and gradually add juice to create a thick dough.

Roll dough out between two pieces of wax paper. Cut out rounds. Place in a dehydrator or in a low oven (200°F) overnight or for 8 hours. Eat within one week.

··· **VARIATIONS** ·······

▶ Sprinkle dough with toasted sesame seeds before cutting.
▶ Use figs in place of dates.
▶ Use lemonade in place of apple or orange juice.

Rainbow Grills

YIELD: 4 servings

PREPARATION TIME: 15 minutes

*Meet your RDA for fruit with this sweet and
healthy dessert or breakfast on a stick.*

1 tablespoon maple syrup

1 teaspoon grated lemon zest

2 teaspoons fresh-squeezed or
   bottled lemon juice

Pinch finely grated nutmeg

1½ pounds assorted fresh fruits
   (such as pineapple, apricots,
   apples, pears, peaches, plums, or
   whole strawberries), halved or
   quartered

Fresh mint sprigs for garnish

Heat oven to 450°F. Cover baking sheet with foil.

Combine all marinade ingredients and set aside.

Thread cubes of fruit on barbecue skewers; use two skewers for each
kebab. Brush with marinade. Place skewers on baking sheet. Roast for 2
minutes; turn and roast again. Repeat, adding marinade while turning.

Serve with plain yogurt or fruit yogurt sauce, garnished with sprigs of
fresh mint.

VARIATIONS

▶ Use agave syrup or honey in place of maple syrup.

▶ Add ½ teaspoon cinnamon to marinade.

Stone Fruit Dessert Soup

YIELD: 4 servings

PREPARATION TIME: 20 minutes, plus 1 hour or more chilling time

Apricots for vitamin A, almonds for
vitamin E—a first-rate first or last course.

½ cup raw almonds

1 cup water or more as needed

1½ pounds apricots, peeled, pitted, and chopped

2 teaspoons peeled and grated fresh gingerroot

¼ cup frozen orange or orange blend juice concentrate

1 tablespoon fresh-squeezed or bottled lemon juice

Fresh mint sprigs for garnish

Chopped almonds for garnish

To make nut cream, place nuts in dry blender or nut grinder, and process into a paste. Combine with water, and blend until smooth. Set aside.

Place apricot pieces and gingerroot in food processor or blender, and process until smooth. Add almond nut cream, juice concentrate, lemon juice, and blend well, adding more water if needed. Taste and adjust seasoning (add a pinch of natural sweetener if needed). Pour soup into a container with tight lid and chill.

Serve garnished with mint and chopped nuts.

··· **VARIATIONS** ··

▶ Substitute peaches for apricots and cashews for almonds.

▶ Stir in ¼ to ½ cup plain yogurt before chilling, for added protein and texture.

Chili-Honeyed Melon

YIELD: 4 servings

PREPARATION TIME: 15 minutes

Pair peppers and melon for more potassium, folate, and vitamin A.

3 tablespoons honey

1 ounce white wine, water, or white tea

1 teaspoon chopped red bell pepper

1 teaspoon chopped yellow bell pepper

1 teaspoon seeded and minced serrano chili pepper

1 tablespoon fresh-squeezed or bottled lime juice

1 tablespoon fresh mint

1 medium cantaloupe or other melon

2 to 3 figs, sliced

Mint sprigs for garnish

Combine honey and wine (or alternative) and cook, stirring, until slightly reduced. Add bell peppers. Set pan aside and cool. Add chili pepper, lime juice, and mint.

Cut melon into slices or other shapes, arrange on platter or dessert dishes, top with figs, and spoon syrup on top.

Garnish with mint sprigs.

··· **VARIATIONS** ···

► Omit chili peppers for a milder taste.

► Substitute dates for figs.

► Use grapefruit or lemon juice in place of lime.

DRINKS

Four-Fruit Ginger Ale

YIELD: 4 servings

PREPARATION TIME: 15 minutes

A low-sugar choice for a summer afternoon. The grape-apple combo sweetens the bite of the ginger-citrus combo.

4 apples, cored and sliced (if not organic, also peel)

1-inch piece fresh gingerroot, peeled and chopped

½ cup seedless grapes

½ lemon, peeled and chopped

½ lime, peeled and chopped

Sparkling mineral water

Blend the apple and gingerroot together; then add the rest of the fruit, and blend again. Pour into four large glasses; fill with sparkling water and ice.

··· **VARIATIONS** ···

▶ Use blueberries in place of grapes.

▶ Omit the lemon, and use sparkling lemon-flavored water in place of plain.

▶ Garnish with mint leaves, or top with a few dried acai berries.

Flavonoid-Filled Limeade

YIELD: 3 to 4 servings
PREPARATION TIME: 15 minutes

Try this low-calorie bioflavonoid-rich soda substitute.

Juice of 3 to 4 limes
2 tablespoons peeled and finely
    grated fresh gingerroot
½ teaspoon liquid stevia, liquid
    honey, or agave syrup, to taste

4 cups filtered water
Orange or lemon slices for garnish

Combine all ingredients with filtered water in a tall pitcher filled with ice cubes. Chill before serving. Garnish with orange or lemon slices.

VARIATION

▶ Substitute 1 cup green tea or mint tea for 1 cup of water.

Soy Smoothie, Six Ways

YIELD: 2 servings

PREPARATION TIME: 5 minutes

A 5-minute nutrition fix from your blender.

1 banana, peeled
½ cup soft silken tofu (about 4 ounces)

2 tablespoons maple syrup or honey
6 ice cubes

Place banana, tofu, maple syrup, and ice in blender, and puree. Pour into two glasses, and serve.

··· **FIVE MORE WAYS** ···

1. **Smoothie Plus:** Add 1 cup fruit juice of your choice and ½ cup fresh or frozen fruit.
2. **Berry-Laced:** Add 1 cup pomegranate-blueberry juice and ½ cup frozen strawberries.
3. **Raspberry:** Add 1 cup orange juice, ½ cup frozen raspberries, and 2 tablespoons lime juice.
4. **Tropical:** Add ¾ cup mango sorbet and 2 tablespoons lime juice.
5. **Cranberry:** Omit maple syrup from base, and add ¾ cup cranberry juice and ½ cup frozen cranberry concentrate.

··· **VARIATIONS** ···

▶ Add antioxidant power with 3 to 4 drops green tea extract.
▶ Add fiber and iron with ¼ cup diced figs or dates.
▶ Add 1 tablespoon flaxseeds for omega-3s.

Anthocyanin Cooler

YIELD: 2 servings

PREPARATION TIME: 10 minutes

Anthocyanins are powerful antioxidants found in the skins of colorful vegetables and fruits such as raspberries, strawberries, and goji berries.

2 dozen fresh large raspberries, divided

6 ounces of seltzer or sparkling water

2 ounces of raw honey or agave syrup

Lemon or green tea ice cubes, crushed

6 ounces of nonalcoholic champagne or sparkling white wine

Mint leaves for garnish

Place all but two of the raspberries in a blender jar with seltzer or sparkling water and honey or syrup. Puree mixture. Fill two chilled glasses with the crushed ice. Divide puree into the two glasses, and top with champagne or white wine. Garnish with fresh mint and reserved raspberries.

VARIATIONS

► Substitute strawberries for raspberries.
► Freeze mint tea to use for ice cubes.
► Top with dried goji berries instead of raspberries.

Vitamin C Colada

YIELD: 2 servings

PREPARATION TIME: 15 minutes

Immunity-boosting vitamin C from four sources.

¼ cup grapefruit juice

¼ cup orange juice

¼ cup pineapple juice

¼ cup herbal red tea such as Red
  Zinger or Rooiboos

Shaved or crushed ice

2 sprigs of fresh rosemary for
  garnish

Orange slices for garnish

Put juices into blender with tea, and blend. Put ice in each glass, and pour in blended mixture. Garnish with rosemary and orange slices.

VARIATIONS

► Substitute 2 or more ounces of coconut milk for herbal tea.

► Garnish with fresh mint in place of rosemary.

► Blend with 1 cup of plain yogurt for a creamier drink.

Spirits-Free Sangria

YIELD: 6 servings

PREPARATION TIME: 10 minutes, plus chilling time

Party in a pitcher with fruit phytonutrients, no buzz!

½ bottle nonalcoholic white wine

¼ cup peach nectar

2 tablespoons sugar or ½ teaspoon stevia

1 tablespoon white grape juice

1 tablespoon fresh-squeezed or bottled lemon juice

½ lemon, sliced

1 medium peach or nectarine, cut into thin wedges

1 cup ice cubes

1 cup chilled sparkling water

Combine wine, nectar, sugar, white grape juice, and lemon juice in a pitcher. Stir well, cover, and chill for at least 1 hour. Add lemon slices and peach or nectarine wedges to pitcher. Add 1 cup ice cubes and sparkling water.

VARIATIONS

▶ Substitute green tea or mint tea ice cubes for plain ice cubes.

▶ Substitute apricots, plums, or kiwi for peaches.

▶ Add ¼ cup of blueberries to pitcher before serving.

Green Ginger Spritzer

YIELD: 3 to 4 servings

PREPARATION TIME: 20 minutes

A high antioxidant alternative to sugary ginger ale.

2 cups prepared green tea

1 bunch green grapes

1 cup sparkling spring water

1-inch piece peeled fresh gingerroot

Fresh mint (optional)

Let tea cool. Place washed and dried grapes on a sheet of foil, and freeze until grapes are solid but not rock-hard.

In a pitcher, pour in green tea and sparkling water. Place ginger in garlic press, and squeeze juice into pitcher. Add sparkling water.

To serve, put a few frozen grapes (an ice cube substitute) into each glass, and pour in sparkler mix. Top (or not) with sprig of mint.

Eat the grapes when the drink is finished.

··· **VARIATIONS** ····

▶ Use mint tea or mint-flavored green tea in place of green tea.

▶ Use lemon or mint-flavored sparkling water in place of plain.

▶ Use ice cubes in place of frozen grapes.

Irish Breakfast Tea Latte

YIELD: 4 servings

PREPARATION TIME: 20 minutes

Switch up your A.M. drink from tea or coffee to a chocolate-enhanced latte.

8 Irish Breakfast tea bags

4 cups filtered water

1 cup soy or dairy milk

½ teaspoon almond extract

½ teaspoon grated dark chocolate or cocoa

Brew a strong tea using water and teabags.

While brewing, heat milk and beat until foamy. Start with cold milk and whisk briskly as the milk is heating. Don't let it boil.

Add extract to tea. Then pour into four cups or glasses, top with foamed milk, and sprinkle on grated chocolate or cocoa.

VARIATIONS

▶ Substitute English Breakfast tea for Irish, or use a decaffeinated version of either.

▶ Omit the almond extract, or use orange extract instead.

Super Immunity Menus

Four weeks of super immunity menus follow. You can make that eight or more by mixing and matching: swapping lunches for dinners and vice versa. For example, swap Monday's lunch for Friday's lunch, or Saturday's dinner for Monday's dinner. Or repeat week one in place of week four, and so on, using suggested variations.

These meals boost immunity across the board. But to further customize them to target a specific immune center or a specific condition, substitute some of the foods recommended for that immune center, where appropriate (see Chapters 1 and 2).

Note: Italicized items indicate recipes included in the recipes section.

Week One

Day One

BREAKFAST
1 cup fresh-squeezed orange or any berry juice
1 scone with *Black-and-Blue Syrup* (page 125)
½ cup scrambled tofu or scrambled eggs
Green or black tea with sliced lemon

SNACK
1 cup *Vitamin C Colada* (page 218) or milk-berry shake

LUNCH
Hot Peanut Dip-and-Dribble Sauce (page 145) with tofu
Bitter Greens Salad (page 152)
Lime-flavored sparkling water

SNACK
1 cup *Bluegrass Chips* (page 139)

DINNER
Zucchini-Pear Summer-Winter Soup (page 166)
Baked yam or sweet potato with whipped tofu topping

Tossed greens with *Pecan-Mint Pesto* (page 144)
Alcohol-free beer

Day Two

BREAKFAST

1 cup whole-grain cereal with steamed apple or pear slices and walnut
   bits or *Cream of Quinoa and Cranberries* (page 123)
1 cup steamed milk or blueberry-leaf tea

LUNCH

Tossed mixed greens with *Fig Vinaigrette* (page 146)
Broiled tempeh burger on whole wheat English muffin with *Black-and-
   Brown Health Hummus* (page 136)
1 slice watermelon or cantaloupe or handful of *Munch-and-Crunch
   Walnuts* (page 205)

SNACK

1 rice cake with *Soy Sour Cream, Three Ways* (page 141) or *Capsaicin
   Salsa* (page 140)

DINNER

Big Bowl Borscht (page 165) with broccoli, alfalfa, or clover sprouts
1 low-fat corn muffin or *Small Potato Chapatis* (page 129)
Chai tea or alcohol-free red wine

Day Three

BREAKFAST

3 broiled pineapple rings or sliced mango with flax sprinkles
1 cup hot oat bran cereal or oat flakes with soy milk or low-fat dairy
   milk
White tea with stevia

SNACK

Moroccan "Caviar" (page 135) or unsalted butter on rice cracker

LUNCH

Veggie burger on whole-grain pita bread or *Sweet Potato Slurpy*
   (page 167)

Tossed greens with *Citrusy Carrot-Ginger Dressing* (page 147)
1 small apple or tangerine or 2 *Drop-Outs* (page 210)
Green-ginger tea

SNACK
Handful of pistachios or mixed nuts

DINNER
Vegetable broth with broccoli or lentil sprouts or *Protein Pea Soup*
    (page 168)
No-Fry Fritters (page 182) or take-out/frozen whole wheat pizza
Steamed or baked squash
1 cup *Chocolate Tofousse* (page 208) or low-sugar chocolate pudding

Day Four

BREAKFAST
1 cup *Pie in a Glass* (pages 200 and 201), either variation, or *Stone Fruit
    Dessert Soup* (page 212)
1 slice nut bread

SNACK
Vegetable sticks with salsa dip or *Olive-Oil Mayonnaise* (page 143)

LUNCH
1 cup *Cream of Wheat Berry Soup* (page 162) or canned organic cream
    of mushroom soup
Rye crackers with garlic butter or *Mustard Greens Pesto* (page 142)
2 sugar-free fig bars

SNACK
1 cup lemon yogurt or *Chai Rice Pudding* (page 209)

DINNER
1 soy dog with *Basil Couscous with Squash* (page 171)
Broiled tomatoes with dairy or nondairy Parmesan cheese
1 cup fruit sorbet with 1 *Beta-Glucan Oatmeal Cookie* (page 198)

Day Five

BREAKFAST

1 cup high-protein cereal (amaranth, quinoa, multigrain) with skim or
   soy milk and sunflower seeds
1 cup pomegranate-blueberry juice or other berry juice

SNACK

1 cup *Flavonoid-Filled Limeade* (page 215) or 2 ounces dried fruit

LUNCH

Pepita Squash Spread (page 134) or guacamole on whole-grain bagel
1 cup tangerine sections or 1 small navel orange
1 cup skim or rice milk

SNACK

1 ounce dark chocolate and 1 cup black or oolong tea

DINNER

Baby spinach salad with *Pink Dressing for Greens* (page 149) or stir-
   fried kale
Parsnip-Ginger Curry (page 185) with steamed brown or basmati rice
2 *Dried-Fruit Truffles* (page 202) or dried dates or figs
Sparkling spring water, plain or flavored

Day Six

BREAKFAST

1 cup pomegranate-berry juice
Flaxberry Flapjacks (page 124) or organic pancakes
Sliced pear or kiwi
Mint tea

SNACK

1 glass kefir or 1 cup yogurt

LUNCH

Raw Slaw 2 (with Kale) (page 155)
Black-and-Brown Health Hummus (page 136) on black bread
Soy Smoothie, Six Ways (page 216), any variation

SNACK
Mixed nuts and seeds or low-salt pretzel rings

DINNER
Fruit and Root Spinach Salad (page 160) or spinach greens salad
Sizzlin' Seitan (page 178) or frozen vegetable lasagna
Brown rice or quinoa
Probiotic Parfait (page 199) or fruit yogurt

Day Seven

BREAKFAST
Fruit salad with yogurt or kefir and flaxseed sprinkles
1 blueberry muffin or *Sweet Potato–Chive Bisquit* (page 128)
Herbal tea, your choice

SNACK
All-natural fruit-and-nut energy bar or 1 cup *Anthocyanin Cooler*
   (page 217)

LUNCH
Marinated Kale Salad (page 153) or mesclun salad with oil-vinegar
   dressing
Miso soup with tofu cubes
Low-fat chocolate milk or soy chocolate milk

SNACK
Sliced peach, nectarine, or orange

DINNER
Watermelon and Tomato Salad (page 151) or baby spinach salad
Wheat Meat Meatballs (page 190) or take-out/frozen meatless
   meatballs
Whole wheat couscous or brown basmati rice
Pinot Noir Pears (page 207) or sliced fresh pear

Week Two

Day One

BREAKFAST
Portobello–Wild Rice Pancakes (page 131) with plain yogurt topping
Peppermint tea or black tea with lemon or orange slices

SNACK
Whole-grain crackers with organic peanut butter

LUNCH
Immunity Toss-Up 1 (page 156) or mesclun salad with sesame-oil
    dressing
Broiled tofu squares or *Purple Potato Colcannon* (page 186)
Whole wheat croissant or ½ whole-grain bagel

SNACK
Low-sodium pretzels and *Spirits-Free Sangria* (page 219)

DINNER
Meatlesss Cacciatore (page 184) or take-out vegetable sushi
Carrot-beet-cabbage slaw with hemp seeds or sesame seeds
½ papaya or ½ cup melon cubes
Ginger-peach tea or juiced tea (half herbal tea, half juice)

Day Two

BREAKFAST
Baked apple or *Rainbow Grills* (page 211)
1 oat bran muffin with omega-3 butter spread
Organic decaf coffee

SNACK
¼ cup goji berries and sunflower seeds or trail mix with berries

LUNCH
Black Bean and Walnut Burger (page 177) with sprouts and shredded
    lettuce or cabbage

1 cup fresh or frozen cherries
Naturally sweetened lemonade

SNACK
½ bagel with low-fat cream cheese or *Edamole* (page 138)

DINNER
Hijiki-Shiitake Sloppy Joe (page 187) or beans and rice
Immunity Toss-Up 2 (page 157) or arugula-leek salad with low-fat
    Green Goddess dressing and toasted dulse
2 *Beta-Glucan Oatmeal Cookies* (page 198) or 1 oatmeal-raisin scone
Alcohol-free beer or wine

Day Three

BREAKFAST
1 poached egg with *Olive-Oil Mayonnaise* (page 143) or *Moroccan
    "Caviar"* (page 135)
1 whole-grain English muffin
1 cup mixed berries, fresh or frozen
Ginger-lemon tea

SNACK
1 *Bellini Brownie* (page 204) and a cup of decaf coffee

LUNCH
Cold rice or couscous salad with shredded carrots, tofu or tempeh
    cubes, and flaxseed-oil dressing
Whole wheat breadsticks or baked chips
½ cup trail mix with dark chocolate bits
Hot or iced black tea

SNACK
1 cup popped popcorn with olive oil and salt-free seasoning or kelp
    powder

DINNER
Chard and Barley Stew (page 179) or frozen veggie burger
Steamed amaranth, couscous, or other whole grain

Power Kraut (page 158) or raw broccoli, celery, and cherry tomatoes
with yogurt dip
1 natural peanut butter cookie
Sparkling spring water on the rocks

Day Four

BREAKFAST
Rosemary and Thyme Frittata (page 194) or scrambled tofu
1 blueberry or date scone
Low-fat hot chocolate

SNACK
1 rice cake with natural peanut or cashew butter

LUNCH
Hijiki Stir-Fry (page 183) or TLT (tofu, lettuce, tomato) on whole wheat
sesame bun with low-sodium pickle
1 fresh apple or fruit cup

SNACK
1 glass low-sodium vegetable juice or fresh-squeezed beet-cucumber-
basil juice

DINNER
Raw Slaw 1 (with Chard) (page 154) or low-fat take-out cole slaw
Immunity Meatloaf (page 191)
Wild rice or quinoa, steamed
Low-sugar soy ice cream

Day Five

BREAKFAST
Spelt flakes with soy or rice milk and dried goji or blueberries
Natural apple or cranberry-apple juice
Handful of mixed nuts

SNACK
2 *Dried-Fruit Truffles* (page 202)

LUNCH
Organic canned lentil soup or *Lentil-Dulse Soup* (page 169)
Sprouted wheat bread or rye roll
Fruit cup or 2 fresh or dried figs or dates

SNACK
Handful of toasted soy nuts or *Edamole* (page 138) on pita bread

DINNER
Red cabbage coleslaw with balsamic vinegar
Multivitamin Moussaka (page 188)
Mashed Potatoes Plus (page 170) or home fries
Alcohol-free red or pink wine
Pie in a Glass (pages 200 and 201), either variation, or fruit sorbet

Day Six

BREAKFAST
Muesli cereal or oat flakes cereal with soy rice or low-fat milk
2 pineapple rings or canned pineapple
Orange-mint tea

SNACK
1 bunch black, green, or red grapes (organic or U.S. grown)

LUNCH
Minted White Gazpacho (page 164) or low-sodium canned gazpacho
Broccoli sprouts or lentil sprouts
1 whole wheat bun or croissant

SNACK
Olives and cubed cheese in extra-virgin olive oil or *Olive-Oil Mayonnaise* (page 143)

DINNER
Spinach-Apple Salad with Maple Dressing (page 150) or watercress salad with walnut oil and walnuts
Blackened Tempeh (page 193) or broiled vegetarian sausage links

Steamed brown rice or couscous
Fresh or frozen berries over plain yogurt

Day Seven

BREAKFAST
Baked apple or broiled red grapefruit half
Rice flakes with rice or soy milk or oatmeal with soy half-and-half
Lemon-green tea

SNACK
Small bunch grapes or banana

LUNCH
Cold beans and rice salad with *Toaster Oven Tomatoes* (page 172)
Spelt bread with omega-3 butter
1 *Beta-Glucan Oatmeal Cookie* (page 198)

SNACK
Papaya Pudding Smoothie (page 206)

DINNER
Miso broth or low-sodium vegetable broth with whole wheat
    croutons
DIY Thai Curry (Raw) (page 181)
Steamed broccoli or *Peanut Butter Broccoli* (page 174)
Peach or passion fruit sorbet

Week Three

Day One

BREAKFAST
Flaxberry Flapjacks (page 124) with plain yogurt topping and sprinkle
    of slivered almonds
Low-sugar hot chocolate or coffee with soy half-and-half (or dairy
    skim milk) and stevia

SNACK
Four-Fruit Ginger Ale (page 214) and 2 to 3 dates or figs

LUNCH
Beta-Carotene Bisque (page 161) or low-sodium vegetable broth with
    steamed carrots
Toasted spelt or whole-grain bread with *Olive-Oil Mayonnaise*
    (page 143)
1 small tangerine or banana

SNACK
Air-popped popcorn or handful of wasabi-spiced nuts

DINNER
Bitter Greens Salad (page 152)
Purple Potato Colcannon (page 186)
1 cornmeal biscuit or corn muffin
Chili-Honeyed Melon (page 213)

Day Two

BREAKFAST
Irish Breakfast Tea Latte (page 221)
1 *Four-Grain Scone* (page 130) or whole wheat croissant with no-sugar
    jelly or jam
Cantaloupe wedges or fruit cocktail

SNACK
Sliced kiwi and green tea

LUNCH
Raw vegetable sticks with *Citrusy Carrot-Ginger Dressing* (page 147)
1 soy hot dog on whole wheat bun with sauerkraut or shredded greens
2 *Beta-Glucan Oatmeal Cookies* (page 198)

SNACK
1 buckwheat rice cake with almond butter

DINNER
Raw Slaw 1 (with Chard) (page 154)
Summer-Squash Pasta with Summer Herbs (page 195)
Probiotic Parfait (page 199) or raspberry soy ice cream
Alcohol-free white wine

Day Three

BREAKFAST
Breakfast Pick-Up Sticks (page 133)
1 navel orange or bunch of organic or U.S.-grown grapes
Ginger-ginseng tea

SNACK
Plain yogurt or kefir with flaxseed sprinkles or sunflower seeds

LUNCH
Spinach-Apple Salad with Maple Dressing (page 150)
Whole wheat sesame breadsticks

SNACK
Pepita Squash Spread (page 134) on mini whole-grain toasted pita
   bread

DINNER
Big Bowl Borscht (page 165) or low-sodium canned beet soup with
   sprouts
Sizzlin' Seitan (page 178)
Basil Couscous with Squash (page 171) or steamed brown rice
Pie in a Glass 2 (page 201)

Day Four

BREAKFAST
Portobello–Wild Rice Pancakes (page 131) with *Miso Vinaigrette*
   (page 148)
Sliced orange or melon
Oolong or black tea

SNACK
1 cup *Soy Smoothie, Six Ways* (page 216), any variation

LUNCH
Minted White Gazpacho (page 164) or cream of mushroom soup from
     salad bar or deli
1 sourdough roll or multigrain roll with omega-3 fortified butter or
     margarine
Ginger-mint tea

SNACK
2 pieces *Health Halvah* (page 203)

DINNER
Fruit and Root Spinach Salad (page 160)
Wheat Meat Meatballs (page 190)
Sesame crackers
Chocolate Tofousse (page 208) or low-fat chocolate (dairy or nondairy)
     ice cream
Alcohol-free wine

Day Five

BREAKFAST
Cream of Quinoa and Cranberries (page 123) or no-sugar granola with
     soy or rice milk
Fresh pineapple or mango slices
Peach-ginger tea or other herbal tea

SNACK
2 ounces trail mix or dried fruit

LUNCH
1 soy hot dog or veggie burger with *Capsaicin Salsa* (page 140)
Baked French fries or oven-baked chips

SNACK
Spirits-Free Sangria (page 219) or naturally sweetened ginger ale with
     gingersnaps

DINNER
Spicy Granny Smith Salad (page 159)
Mashed Potatoes Plus (page 170)
No-Fry Fritters (page 182)
1 slice pound cake or 3 *Dried-Fruit Truffles* (page 202)
Sparkling mineral water

Day Six

BREAKFAST
Oatmeal with toasted walnuts and a swirl of yogurt
Irish Breakfast Tea Latte (page 221) or black tea

SNACK
Flavonoid-Filled Limeade (page 215) or low-sugar lemonade

LUNCH
1 *Black Bean and Walnut Burger* (page 177) on multigrain bread
Marinated Kale Salad (page 153) or baby greens with balsamic vinegar
1 banana or sliced papaya

SNACK
1 oatmeal muffin with omega-3-fortified margarine or butter

DINNER
Peas Twice (page 173)
Better Red Risotto (page 180)
Whole-grain bagel slices, toasted
Pinot Noir Pears (page 207) or baked apple

Day Seven

BREAKFAST
Seven-grain cereal with soy, rice, or dairy milk and toasted flaxseed
½ small melon or pineapple rings
White or green tea

SNACK
1 cup air-popped popcorn or *Cumin-Spiced Popcorn* (page 137)

LUNCH
Cashew nut butter and jelly sandwich on whole-grain bread
Raw Slaw 1 (with Chard) (page 154)
1 large organic apple or ½ cup sugar-free applesauce

SNACK
Yogurt or kefir, plain or with fruit

DINNER
Peanut Butter Broccoli (page 174)
Soy-sauce-broiled tempeh or tofu
Soy Succotash (page 176)
Pie in a Glass 2 (page 201) or *Chili-Honeyed Melon* (page 213)

Week Four

Day One

BREAKFAST
Oat, Kamut, or multigrain flakes with fresh or dried blueberries or
    cranberries
Oat, soy, rice, or low-fat dairy milk
Oolong or jasmine tea with stevia

SNACK
½ cup baked corn chips or potato chips or handful of mini pretzels

LUNCH
Mixed leafy greens with *Citrusy Carrot-Ginger Dressing* (page 147)
1 *Four-Grain Scone* (page 130) with *Olive-Oil Mayonnaise* (page 143)
Darjeeling tea with honey and lemon

SNACK
Mini box unsulphured raisins or banana

DINNER
Bitter Greens Salad (page 152) or baby spinach salad
Blackened Tempeh (page 193) or frozen veggie burger
Basil Couscous with Squash (page 171)
Chili-Honeyed Melon (page 213)
Chamomile tea or decaf coffee

Day Two

BREAKFAST
1 honey-baked apple or pear or *Breakfast Bruschetta* (page 126)
Handful of raw nuts and seeds
Coffee or café Americano (half coffee, half steamed milk)

SNACK
1 toasted rice cake with *Capsaicin Salsa* (page 140) or store-bought salsa

LUNCH
Romaine lettuce with *Mustard Greens Pesto* (page 142)
1 grilled cheese (or vegetarian cheese) sandwich on whole wheat bread
Fresh fruit cocktail

SNACK
Handful of organic or U.S.-grown grapes, red or green

DINNER
Coleslaw with balsamic or rice wine vinegar
Cream of Wheat Berry Soup (page 162)
1 sourdough roll with extra-virgin olive oil or flaxseed oil
1 cup canned (in water) peaches or fresh fruit salad
Sparkling mineral water or *Spirits-Free Sangria* (page 219)

Day Three

BREAKFAST
Breakfast Berry Pops (page 132)
1 toasted whole-grain croissant
Black tea or iced black tea with stevia or raw honey

SNACK
6 mini pretzels and *Green Ginger Spritzer* (page 220)

LUNCH
Black-and-Brown Health Hummus (page 136) on seven-grain bread or
    whole-grain crackers
Bitter Greens Salad (page 152)
Juiced tea (half herbal tea, half juice)

DINNER
Peas Twice (page 173)
1 *Hoppin' John Burger* (page 196) with steamed brown rice or quinoa, or
    veggie burger
Soy Smoothie, Six Ways (page 216), any variation, or *Probiotic Parfait*
    (page 199)

Day Four

BREAKFAST
Frozen whole-grain waffles with *Black-and-Blue Syrup* (page 125)
Sliced banana or frozen blackberries
Oolong or jasmine tea

SNACK
2 pieces *Health Halvah* (page 203)

LUNCH
Big Bowl Borscht (page 165) with tofu "croutons" or tomato soup from
    deli
Marinated Kale Salad (page 153)
Dry-roasted pistachio nuts

SNACK
Pepita Squash Spread (page 134) on rice cakes or rye crackers

DINNER
Raw vegetables with *Soy Sour Cream, Three Ways* (page 141), any
    variation
Chard and Barley Stew (page 179)

Sesame breadsticks
Probiotic Parfait (page 199)

Day Five

BREAKFAST
Cream of Quinoa and Cranberries (page 123) with flaxseed sprinkles
    and scoop of yogurt
Irish Breakfast Tea Latte (page 221) or black tea

SNACK
Bunch of grapes, organic or U.S. grown

LUNCH
Spicy Granny Smith Salad (page 159) or apple-cabbage coleslaw
1 *Four-Grain Scone* (page 130) or whole wheat croissant or bagel
Alcohol-free beer

SNACK
Cumin-Spiced Popcorn (page 137) or trail mix

DINNER
Watermelon and Tomato Salad (page 151)
Spicy Tofu Minute Steaks (page 192) or broiled tofu
Mashed Potatoes Plus (page 170) or oven-baked fries
Chocolate Tofousse (page 208)

Day Six

BREAKFAST
Scrambled eggs or scrambled tofu
1 slice nut bread
Green Ginger Spritzer (page 220)

SNACK
2 to 3 pieces *Health Halvah* (page 203)

LUNCH
Raw Slaw 1 (with Chard) (page 154) or *Raw Slaw 2 (with Kale)* (page 155)

1 soy hot dog with *Capsaicin Salsa* (page 140) on whole wheat bun
1 *Beta-Glucan Oatmeal Cookie* (page 198) or oat scone

SNACK
1 cup grape juice, red or white

DINNER
Peas Twice (page 173)
Parsnip-Ginger Curry (page 185)
Basil Couscous with Squash (page 171) or steamed brown basmati rice
Sesame crackers
Fruit sorbet or *Pinot Noir Pears* (page 207)

Day Seven

BREAKFAST
Breakfast Pick-Up Sticks (page 133)
Sliced peach or banana
Fruit juice or juiced tea (half herbal tea, half juice)

SNACK
Mixed raw nuts

LUNCH
Pink Roasted Beets (page 175) or beet salad
1 grilled cheese (dairy or nondairy cheese) sandwich on whole-grain
    bread with sprouts
½ cup baked corn chips or potato chips
Sparkling water

SNACK
2 natural butter cookies

DINNER
1 *Hijiki-Shiitake Sloppy Joe* (page 187)
Steamed millet or rice
Soy Succotash (page 176)
Alcohol-free wine
Sliced papaya or peach

Putting It All Together: Super Immunity Foods in Action

You know the twenty-five immunity boosters and thirteen busters, and you've got a month's worth of menus and recipes, plus dozens of culinary and nutritional kitchen tips. To create lifelong immunity, for starters, research indicates, you will add an average of fourteen years to your life span if you do just four things:

1. Eat lots of fruits and vegetables.
2. Don't smoke.
3. Exercise.
4. Drink alcohol in moderation.

You'll add even *more* days and *more* quality of life if you add the following twenty-nine strategies to those four steps.

At the Table, in the Kitchen

▶ **Eat more (but not all) food raw.** Having five to nine ½ cup servings of fruits and vegetables daily, most raw and from the SIF (Super Immunity Foods) roster, can boost your immunity, especially to cancer, heart disease, obesity, and diabetes.

▶ **Five signs that a food is a good immune booster?** It's richly colored, it's fresh, it's organically grown, it's in season, and it's locally produced. (Three out of five is good, too.) What qualifies? Think of fresh unsprayed strawberries in June, just-picked corn in July, locally grown tomatoes in August, and just-dug potatoes from somewhere in-state. Some next-best choices? Organic but frozen spinach, local but nonorganic squash, and fresh and sustainably grown but not local peas and carrots.

▶ **Support local farmers.** Go to the local green market on the weekend, or join a community-supported agriculture (CSA) and get regular deliveries of in-season produce from the farmer around the block or in the next county. To find out who's where, go to localharvest.org/csa. During the week, do your own small-scale farming, and grow your favorite herbs or miniature vegetables on your windowsill or back patio. If you've got a back forty, put an inexpensive inflatable greenhouse in it.

▶ **Eat organically *and* locally when you can.** Organic fruits and vegetables from a farm near you can provide up to 59 percent higher levels of antioxidants than their conventionally grown counterparts, says the Organic Consumers Association. If you can't eat organic all the time, make sure you eat these twelve foods from the organic aisle: apples, apricots, bell peppers, cantaloupe, celery, cherries, cucumbers, green beans, peaches, spinach, strawberries, and grapes. Grapes from the United States are OK, but pass up the imported grapes.

▶ **Protect your children's plates.** In one study by the Environmental Working Group, children who ate conventional produce and juice had six to nine times more pesticide residue in their bodies than children who ate organically. Pesticides can damage the nervous and hormonal systems as well as the thyroid gland. Cook less, and steam, boil, or stir-fry when you do. Acrylamide, a carcinogen, is formed when frying, baking, or grilling at high temperatures. When you do heat things up, small changes matter. Adding rosemary to your baked goods, for example, can reduce the cancer risk by up to 60 percent. And adding blueberries to meat (if you eat it) does the same.

▶ **Juice daily.** It's a great way to get and even exceed your five to nine servings of fruits and vegetables daily. According to studies at the Federal Research Centre for Nutrition and Food in Germany, drinking 12 ounces of either carrot or tomato juice (both rich in carotenoids) caused a jump in natural killer (NK) immune cell activity in the blood by 25 percent.

▶ **Let color be your guide for super immunity.** Half the vegetables you eat should be red or orange; the other half should be dark green, blue, and black. But save space for those white potatoes and mushrooms, too.

▶ **Have small meals taken often.** The larger the meal, the more stress you generate for the organs of digestion and detoxification. Having six small nutritionally dense meals daily is ideal.

▶ **Supplement smart.** Compensate for nutrients depleted by any prescription medications you are on (see naturalnews.com/drug watch_home.html for a list) as well as those lost due to illness or medical conditions. A good diet alone doesn't cover all the bases anymore.

▶ **Eat yogurt or kefir daily.** As much as 60 percent of your immune cells are located in your gut. If you miss, take a quality probiotic supplement.

▶ **Consider the senses.** Add crunchy, hot or cold, and colorful to every meal to satisfy the senses, boost nutrition, and reduce the risk of overeating. For example, add a tablespoon of crunchy cereal to a bowl of hot oatmeal, arrange colorful steamed vegetables alongside a cold sandwich, and add crisp nuts to a smooth pasta sauce.

▶ **Calculate your sugar intake.** Sugar lowers your immunity. There are better, safer substitutes to keep your coffee sweet and your sugar bowl filled. Try the zero-calorie herbal sugar, stevia, in powder or liquid form, or Sun Crystals, a combination of raw sugar and erythritol formulated from non-GMO fruits and vegetables at 4 calories a packet. For baking, use raw honey, maple syrup, agave syrup, or brown rice syrup—all in moderation.

▶ **Monitor your caffeine intake.** This stimulant found in coffee, regular tea, chocolate, some soft drinks, and over-the-counter drugs (e.g., some antihistamine formulas) not only negatively impacts your blood pressure, bladder, and kidneys as well as blood sugar levels but also can deplete calcium and cause dehydration if you overdo it, especially in the already "underwatered" among us. Too much may also up- or down-regulate your appetite.

▶ **Keep your sweet tooth happy and healthy.** Keep bits of candied ginger, dark chocolate, and dried berries in the candy jar.

▶ **Keep a healthy pH balance.** A key measure of your overall health is your acid-alkaline balance, expressed as a number on the pH scale: 1 is most acid and 14 is most alkaline. You can check your numbers (excellent is between 6.6 and 6.8) with a litmus paper test kit available from medical supply companies or some health pharmacies.

▶ **Toss a leafy green salad, and toss it off daily at lunch, dinner, breakfast, or even in between meals.** Add garlic or onions every time.

▶ **Drink tea.** Aim for two cups or more; hot or iced; black, green, or oolong. Having a third? Make it herbal.

▶ **Once-a-day nuts.** Have a handful of nuts (unroasted, unsalted) between meals every day.

▶ **Put plastic aside.** Polyvinyl chloride used in cling wraps and flexible water bottles is a source of phthalates linked to reproductive damage, while polycarbonate used in water jugs, baby bottles, and as a lining in aluminum cans can leach bisphenol A, an estrogenic compound linked to breast cancer and an increased risk of diabetes. Polypropylene used in plastic storage containers can also leach dangerous toxins into foods when heated. All plastics pose a danger to marine life and the environment at large. Switch to Pyrex or stoneware, and go back to old-fashioned wax paper.

▶ **Buy only what you can eat and waste not.** The average American family discards 122 pounds of food each month. That rotting food that ends up in landfills produces methane, a major contributor to greenhouse gases. Worse, recovering just 5 percent of the food that is wasted could feed 4 million people a day. Make it 25 percent, and 20 million people who are starving wouldn't.

Away from the Table

▶ **Frequent driver?** Get an air cleaner for your backseat. Dirty air contributes to everything from lung disease to low birth weight. Driving or jogging along heavily trafficked highways is hazardous. Breathing in particulates, nitrogen oxides, benzenes, and other air pollutants can increase your risk of dying from heart failure and respiratory disease. Pollution contributes to the hardening of the arteries, abnormal heart rhythms, even the thickening of the blood, according to a report commissioned by the Environmental Protection Agency in 2004.

▶ **Don't pump your own gas.** If you do, find a pump with a fume-diffusing nozzle and look away. The benzene in gasoline is an immunity-depleting toxin, also found in some commercial household cleaning products. Switch to all-green cleaning products.

▶ **Snooze on schedule.** Sleep deprivation can increase your C-reactive protein (CRP) levels fivefold, indicate some studies. Worse, sleeplessness becomes a pattern remedied with pharmaceuticals that, in the long run, compound the problem by generating more toxins and creating dependency.

▶ **Think pharmokinetically.** All prescription drugs deplete essential nutrients, commonly B vitamins, folate, vitamin C, calcium, and magnesium. All statin drugs deplete coenzyme Q_{10}, which is critical for normal heart function and energy. Even ordinary aspirin depletes vitamin C, folate, potassium, iron, and sodium. Don't take drugs that you don't need. More than 100,000 people die annually of side effects from prescription drugs (twenty times the number of deaths from illegal drugs).

▶ **Take breaths.** Learn to breathe deeply. Breathing in the typical shallow-chested way keeps your lungs underexercised, deprives you of the rewards of fully oxygenating your brain and all the body's tissues, and keeps stress locked into your joints and organs. Watch a video or take a workshop on Yogic breathing (*pranayama*). Aerobic activities also force you to use your respiratory system optimally.

▶ **Zone out and bond.** Get a grip on your emotions. Negative feelings set off alarms in all of the immune centers (especially those where you are most vulnerable). Develop give-and-take relationships you can fall back on, even if it's just your bridge partner and your dutiful dachshund.

▶ **What's on your lawn?** Whatever it is, it's also on your shoes, on your rugs, and in your lungs—and it could be toxic to your immune system. Explore natural alternatives to pest and weed control.

▶ **Monitor your TV time.** Viewing more than two hours a day elevates your risk of obesity, Metabolic Syndrome, and cardiovascular disease. Unless you're meditating, sit less.

▶ **Drink responsibly, if at all.** Switch to alcohol-free wines and beers. Alcohol can interfere with the absorption of the very nutrients you're taking to protect yourself from the diseases that result when your immunity is low. You want to create virtuous, not vicious, circles with your choices.

Resources

Sources

Sea Vegetables
www.seaveg.com
www.seaweed.net

Stevia Herbal Sweetener
www.stevitastevia.com

Heirloom Seeds
www.seedsavers.org
www.heirloomseeds.com

Yogurt Makers
www.yogurtnet.com

Sprouting Seeds and Kits
www.sproutpeople.com

Dried Berries, Exotic Fruit
www.friedas.com
www.melissas.com

Heirloom Apples
www.localharvest.org

Portable Greenhouses
www.allgreenhouses.com

Wheat Grass, Seeds, and Juicers
www.wheatgrasskits.com

Nutritional Supplements
www.invitehealth.com

Liquid Aminos
www.bragg.com

Organizations

The Cancer Project
www.CancerProject.org

Physicians Committee for Responsible Medicine
www.pcrm.org

Index

Page numbers in **boldface** indicate recipes.